MW00884866

THE

OSTEOPOROSIS-FREE

LIFESTYLE

A Complete Healthy Diet Plan for Stronger Joints and Bones

© 2024 by Marilyn S. Humble

All rights reserved. No part of this publication may be reproduced, distributed, or transmitted in any form or by any means, including photocopying, recording, or other electronic or mechanical methods, without the prior written permission of the publisher, except in the case of brief quotations embodied in critical reviews and certain other noncommercial uses permitted by copyright law.

TABLE OF CONTENT

INTRODUCTION

Remembering my Aunt Margaret and Uncle Joe always makes me realize how important it is to take care of my bones. Their shared story spans over half a century and exemplifies the ways in which osteoporosis affects everyday life and the power of positive decision-making.

The first member of our family to get an osteoporosis diagnosis was Aunt Margaret. We still talk about the day she heard the news. She had just fallen, describing it as a little slip on a damp bathroom floor; she was in her early sixties. Nevertheless, she endured unbearable hip discomfort and, after seeing a doctor, learned the worst: she had a fracture, the result of bones that had become dangerously brittle. It was hard to imagine that this vivacious lady, who had always been the foundation of our family, suddenly faced a future of uncertainty and physical limits. Her life was drastically altered by the diagnosis.

Out of nowhere, routine chores turned into insurmountable obstacles. For fear of injuring herself further in another fall, she was anxious about every step she made. Sturdy Uncle Joe, who had previously guarded Margaret, now found himself in the position of her continual companion and caretaker. Watching children adjust to this new reality was both upsetting and eye-opening for our whole family.

But it wasn't until Uncle Joe's own diagnosis of osteoporosis a few years later that I fully started to comprehend the significance of this hidden illness. Joe had always been robust and tough, the type of guy who seldom saw a doctor. When his back discomfort began, he put it up to old age and years of hard labor. It wasn't until he could no longer ignore the agony that he sought medical help. The diagnosis was another blow—osteoporosis had now crept into his life, threatening to take away the freedom he had always treasured.

So what is osteoporosis, this quiet thief that may so simply suck away the quality of life? Simply defined, it's a disorder where bones grow weak and brittle, leaving them more prone to fractures. For many, like Aunt Margaret and Uncle Joe, it comes as a surprise—something that happens to "other people," not to them. Yet osteoporosis affects millions, especially as people age, and the indicators might be modest at first. A fracture after a slight fall, chronic back discomfort, a loss of height—these are the early warning symptoms that sometimes go unrecognized until the harm is done.

Understanding osteoporosis is the first step in avoiding it. The problem develops when the development of new bone doesn't keep up with the elimination of old bone. This imbalance may be altered by several variables, including age, gender, family history, and lifestyle choices. Women, particularly those post-menopause, are at increased risk because of the dramatic reduction in estrogen, a hormone that helps preserve bone density. But males, as Uncle Joe realized, are not immune. Genetics have a role too, as does nutrition, activity, and even how much sunshine you receive.

The consequence of osteoporosis extends well beyond the physical. It may rob away confidence, independence, and the basic pleasures of life. Yet, as I've seen with my family, it doesn't have to be this way. There is a way to stronger bones, one that may help prevent osteoporosis or halt its progression—and it begins with a dedication to a better lifestyle.

This book provides a guide to the Osteoporosis-Free Lifestyle, a method that unifies the fundamental pillars of bone health: diet, activity, and general well-being. The relationship between food and bone health is significant. The nutrients we consume supply the building blocks our bodies require to sustain healthy bones. It's about more than simply calcium—though that's vital too. It's about a balanced diet rich in vitamins and minerals that promote bone density, combined with regular physical exercise that keeps bones strong and joints flexible.

But diet and exercise alone aren't enough. A genuine osteoporosis-free lifestyle entails establishing realistic objectives and implementing permanent adjustments. It's about knowing your body's demands, identifying risk factors, and taking proactive efforts to safeguard your bone health at every stage of life. Whether you're in your twenties, establishing the foundation for strong bones, or in your sixties, like Aunt Margaret, striving to maintain what you have, this strategy may let you enjoy life fully, without the continuous concern of fractures and falls.

Aunt Margaret and Uncle Joe's experiences were a wake-up call for me and our family. We discovered that bone health isn't something to take for granted. It's something to be fostered, safeguarded, and actively maintained. The Osteoporosis-Free Lifestyle is about empowerment—taking responsibility for your health and adopting choices that encourage stronger, healthier bones.

In the chapters that follow, we'll examine what it means to live this lifestyle, from the meals that should fill your plate to the workouts that will keep your bones strong. We'll speak about creating goals, making changes that stay, and finding pleasure in the process. My aim is that this book will serve as a guide to a life free from the limits of osteoporosis, so you may move ahead with confidence, strength, and peace of mind.

1: Nutrition Essentials for Bone Health

The Building Blocks of Strong Bones

The Calcium Role: Not Just in Dairy

Calcium plays a crucial role in maintaining the strength and structure of bone tissue. There are a few other foods that may increase your intake of calcium in addition to dairy products like milk, cheese, and yogurt. Leafy greens (like kale and broccoli), nuts (like almonds), seeds (like chia and sesame), and fortified foods (like plant-based milks and orange juice) are examples of non-dairy calcium sources. Maintaining appropriate calcium levels is essential to prevent the body from losing calcium reserves in the bones, and eating a wide variety of these foods may help achieve this.

Sun Exposure and Vitamin D: Their Significance

Because it enhances stomach calcium absorption and aids in maintaining appropriate blood calcium and phosphate concentrations—both necessary for healthy bone mineralization—vitamin D is crucial for bone health. Sun exposure is essential for bone health because it causes the body to synthesize vitamin D when skin is exposed to sunshine. But fortified foods (like milk and cereals), supplements, and fatty fish (like salmon and mackerel) can also help ensure that vitamin D levels are adequate, especially for people who don't get much sun exposure.

Magnesium, Phosphorus, and Additional Vital Minerals

The active form of vitamin D is converted by magnesium, which improves the absorption of calcium. Nuts, seeds, whole grains, and green leafy vegetables are foods high in magnesium. By neutralizing bone-depleting metabolic acids, potassium helps to keep calcium in the bones. Sweet potatoes, beans, and bananas are rich sources of potassium. Zinc, which is present in meat, seafood, legumes, and seeds, and phosphorus, which is found in protein-rich foods like dairy and meat, are additional essential elements for bone health.

The Power of Protein in Bone Health

Protein is an essential component of bone tissue, required for maintaining bone density and strength. Adequate protein consumption promotes the formation of collagen, which serves as the structural underpinning for bones. Lean meats, poultry, fish, eggs, dairy products, legumes, nuts, and seeds are all excellent sources of protein. Protein consumption must be balanced with other nutrients, since too much protein without enough calcium might cause calcium loss from the bones.

Superfoods for Stronger Bones and Joints

Top 10 Bone-Boosting Foods

1. Dairy Products: Milk, cheese, and yogurt are rich in calcium and vitamin D.
2. Leafy Greens: Kale, spinach, and broccoli offer calcium, magnesium, and vitamin K.
3. Fatty Fish: Salmon, mackerel, and sardines provide high quantities of vitamin D and omega-3 fatty acids.
4. Nuts and Seeds: Almonds, chia seeds, and sesame seeds all include calcium, magnesium, and healthy fats.
5. Fortified Foods: Plant-based milks, orange juice, and cereals typically contain calcium and vitamin D.
6. Beans and Lentils: These legumes are high in calcium, magnesium, and protein.
7. Tofu and Tempeh: Soybeans are excellent plant-based providers of calcium and protein.
8. Fruits: Oranges, figs, and prunes include calcium, potassium, and vitamin C.
9. Whole Grains: Oatmeal, quinoa, and brown rice all contain magnesium and phosphorus.
10. Eggs: An excellent source of vitamin D and protein.

Anti-inflammatory Foods for Joint Health

1) Berries: Blueberries, strawberries, and raspberries are rich in antioxidants and vitamin C.
2) Fatty Fish: High in omega-3 fatty acids, which help decrease inflammation.
3) Olive Oil contains oleocanthal, which has anti-inflammatory qualities.
4) Nuts and Seeds: Rich in omega-3 fatty acids are walnuts, flaxseeds, and chia seeds.
5) Leafy Greens: Rich in vitamins and antioxidants are spinach, kale, and Swiss chard.
6) The powerful anti-inflammatory compound curcumin is found in turmeric.
7) Ginger is well-known for its antioxidant and anti-inflammatory qualities
8) Diallyl disulfide, found in garlic, has anti-inflammatory properties.
9) Green Tea contains polyphenols, which have anti-inflammatory properties.

10) Tomatoes are high in lycopene, an antioxidant with anti-inflammatory qualities.

The Best Plant-Based Sources of Calcium

1. Leafy Greens include kale, collard greens, and bok choy.
2. Fortified Plant Milks: Almond, soybean, and rice milk.
3. Tofu and Tempeh, particularly when cooked with calcium sulfate.
4. Nuts and Seeds include almonds, chia seeds, and sesame seeds.
5. Beans and Lentils: White, chickpeas, and black-eyed peas.
6. Fortified Cereals: Many morning cereals include calcium.
7. Fruits include oranges, figs, and dried apricots.
8. Seaweed, particularly wakame and kelp.
9. Amaranth and Quinoa: Ancient calcium-rich cereals.
10. Broccoli and Brussels sprouts are cruciferous vegetables high in calcium.

Adding Bone-Building Superfoods to Your Diet

1. Breakfast: Start the day with a glass of fortified plant milk and some porridge or cereal that has been fortified. Top with nuts and seeds.
2. Lunch: Have a salad with lemon juice, olive oil, and sesame seeds along with leafy greens.
3. Snack: Indulge in a smoothie made with spinach, berries, and fortified plant milk, or a handful of almonds.
4. Dinner: Serve quinoa and steamed broccoli with fatty fish, such as salmon.
5. Dessert: Serve a fruit salad with oranges, figs, and honey.
6. Supplements: If you get little sun, consider taking a vitamin D supplement, especially if you don't get enough calcium from your diet.

Foods to Avoid for Optimal Bone Health

The Effects of Caffeine, Alcohol, and Sugar

- Caffeine: While moderate caffeine use is normally safe, high intake might impair calcium absorption and cause bone loss. To reduce the influence of caffeine on bone health, restrict your daily consumption to less than 400 mg (approximately four cups of coffee).
- Alcohol: Excessive alcohol use may upset the calcium balance in the body and interfere with the formation of vitamin D, which is required for calcium absorption. Chronic excessive drinking may cause bone loss and raise the risk of fractures. It is preferable to take alcohol in moderation, with a maximum of one drink per day for women and two for males.

- Sugar: A high sugar consumption might cause increased calcium excretion and decreased bone density. Sugary meals and beverages may also contribute to weight growth, placing additional pressure on bones and joints. Cutting down on sugary meals, beverages, and sweets can help you maintain healthy bone health.

Processed food and bone density

Processed meals often include high quantities of salt, harmful fats, and chemicals that may harm bone health. High salt consumption may lead to calcium loss via urine, weakening bones over time. Furthermore, processed meals are often lacking in key elements such as calcium, magnesium, and vitamin D. To promote bone health, restrict your consumption of processed meals and choose whole, nutrient-dense foods.

Balancing Acidic and Alkaline Food

Bone health may be influenced by the body's pH balance. High-acid diets (such as meat, dairy, and processed foods) may cause calcium to be leached from bones in order to neutralize the acid. On the other side, alkaline foods (such as fruits, vegetables, and nuts) may assist maintain a good pH balance and promote bone health. Maintaining a balanced diet rich in alkaline foods may help preserve bone density.

Identifying and managing food sensitivities

Food intolerances and sensitivities may affect overall health, particularly bone health, and the absorption of nutrients. Among the most frequent culprits are dairy, gluten, and certain additives. Consult a medical professional for a diagnosis and treatment if you believe you may have a food sensitivity. Making the necessary food substitutions and doing away with troublesome meals can guarantee that you get the nutrients your body needs for strong bones.

2: Crafting your Osteoporosis-free Diet Plan

The Foundations of a Bone-Healthy Diet

Planning Meals to Build Strong Bones

A diet plan that promotes bone health must include a range of foods high in nutrients that provide vital vitamins and minerals. Make it a goal to include foods high in protein, calcium, magnesium, and vitamin D into your regular meals. A well-rounded meal might consist of a side of fruit and enriched cereal with almond milk. For lunch, you may have a healthy green salad with beans and almonds on top, and for supper, you might have grilled salmon served with quinoa and steamed broccoli. A handful of nuts, cheese, or yogurt are examples of snacks that might increase your daily intake of nutrients.

Moderate Portion Size and Well-Eaten Food

Because being underweight increases the risk of bone loss and fractures, maintaining a healthy weight is essential for bone health. Portion management makes sure you don't overeat while yet consuming the proper quantity of nutrients. Whole foods should be the main focus of a balanced meal, which should also include a variety of healthy fats, carbs, and proteins. You may efficiently control your intake by using smaller dishes, monitoring quantities, and paying attention to serving sizes.

The Vital Significance of Hydration for Healthy Bones

It's essential to stay hydrated for general health, which includes bone health. Water flushes out waste and aids in the transportation of nutrients to your bones. Dehydration raises the risk of fractures and lowers bone density. Try to consume 8 glasses of water or more if you live in a hot area or are physically active each day. Maintaining hydration levels may also be facilitated by including foods high in water, such as fruits and vegetables, in your diet.

BREAKFAST AND BRUNCH

Cottage Cheese with Pineapple

(per serving):

Prep Time: 5 minutes Cooking Time: None

Serving Size: 1 bowl about 1 1/2 cups

Calories**: 220

Protein**: 18g

Fat**: 4g

Carbs: 26g

Fiber: 4g

Calcium: 200 mg

1 cup low-fat cottage cheese

1/2 cup fresh pineapple chunks or canned in its own juice, drained

1 tablespoon chia seeds

1 teaspoon honey

1/4 teaspoon cinnamon

Chop the fresh pineapple into bite-sized pieces if using it.

Put the cottage cheese and pineapple pieces in a bowl. Gently stir to combine.

Garnish with chia seeds, drizzle with honey, and, if you'd like, a dash of cinnamon.

Eat right now, or chill if making ahead.

Whole Wheat Waffles with Greek Yogurt

Prep Time: 10 minutes Cooking Time: 10 minutes

(per serving, 1 waffle with toppings):

Calories: 280

Protein: 12g

Fat: 10g

Carbs: 40g

Fiber: 6g

Calcium: 200 mg

1 cup whole wheat flour

1 tablespoon baking powder

1/2 teaspoon cinnamon (optional)

1 tablespoon honey or maple syrup

1 large egg

1 cup low-fat milk

2 tablespoons olive oil or melted butter

1/2 teaspoon vanilla extract

Toppings:

1/2 cup plain Greek yogurt

1/2 cup fresh mixed fruit (berries, banana slices, or any fruit of choice)

1 tablespoon chia seeds

Drizzle of honey or maple syrup (optional)

Warm up your waffle maker.

Combine the whole wheat flour, baking powder, and cinnamon (if using) in a large basin.

Beat the egg and combine it with the milk, honey, butter, or olive oil in another dish. Add the vanilla essence.

Don't overmix; instead, whisk only until the wet and dry components are incorporated.

Transfer the batter to the waffle iron that has been warmed, and cook it as directed by the maker until it becomes golden and crisp.

Top each waffle with a dollop of Greek yogurt, chia seeds, fresh fruit, and, if preferred, a drizzle of syrup or honey.

Ricotta and Berry Toast on Whole Grain Bread

(per serving, 2 slices):

Calories: 250

Protein: 10g

Fat: 7g

Carbs: 35g

Fiber: 6g

Calcium: 150 mg

Prep Time: 5 minutes Cooking Time: 2 minutes

2 slices whole grain bread

1/4 cup part-skim ricotta cheese

1/2 cup mixed fresh berries

1 teaspoon honey

1/4 teaspoon cinnamon

Until golden brown, lightly toast the whole grain bread.

Evenly cover each piece of bread with ricotta cheese.

Spoon the ricotta over the fresh berries.

If desired, sprinkle cinnamon over top and drizzle with honey.

Spinach and Feta Omelette

(per serving, 1 omelet):

Calories: 260

Protein: 15g

Fat: 21g

Carbs: 3g

Fiber: 1g

Calcium: 250 mg

Prep Time: 5 minutes Cooking Time: 5 minutes

2 large eggs

1/4 cup crumbled feta cheese

1 cup fresh spinach (roughly chopped)

1 tablespoon olive oil or butter

Salt and pepper

A pinch of dried oregano or fresh
herbs

Clean and finely cut the spinach. Put aside.

In a nonstick pan set over medium heat, warm the olive oil. Add the spinach and heat, stirring periodically, for one to two minutes, or until the spinach wilts. Take out of the pan and place aside.

Beat the eggs together with a dash of pepper and salt in a bowl.

Pour the whisked eggs into the same pan, stirring to uniformly coat the bottom. Cook until the edges begin to set, one to two minutes.

Distribute equally over half of the omelet the cooked spinach and crumbled feta cheese.

Fold the omelet in half, cover, and continue cooking for an additional one to two minutes, or until the cheese has melted somewhat and the eggs are well cooked. Warm up and serve.

Tofu Scramble with Spinach

(per serving):

Serving Size: 1 bowl (about 1 1/2 cups)

Prep Time: 5 minutes Cooking Time: 10 minutes

Calories: 220

Protein: 18g

Fat: 12g

Carbs: 8g

Fiber: 4g

Calcium: 300 mg

1 block (14 oz) firm tofu, drained and crumbled

1 tablespoon olive oil

1/2 onion, finely chopped

1 clove garlic, minced

1/2 teaspoon turmeric

1/4 teaspoon ground cumin

2 cups fresh spinach, chopped

Salt and pepper to taste

1 tablespoon nutritional yeast

1/4 cup diced tomatoes or bell peppers

Using a fork or your hands, crush the tofu into tiny pieces after draining it.

In a big pan set over medium heat, warm up the olive oil. Add the minced garlic and onion, and sauté for three to four minutes, or until softened.

To bring out the flavors, stir in the cumin and turmeric and simmer for one minute.

Include the tofu that has crumbled into the skillet. For five to seven minutes, or until the tofu is fully cooked and beginning to turn brown, stir well to coat it with the spices.

Cook the fresh spinach for a further two to three minutes, or until it wilts.

Add nutritional yeast or chopped tomatoes, if preferred, and season with salt and pepper. Warm up and serve.

Salmon and Avocado on Whole-Grain Toast

(per serving):

Serving Size: 2 slices of toast with toppings

Calories: 350

Protein: 20g

Fat: 18g

Carbs: 28g

Fiber: 6g

Calcium: 100 mg

Prep Time: 5 minutes Cooking Time: 5 minutes

2 slices whole-grain bread, toasted

1/2 ripe avocado

1/2 cup cooked salmon (fresh or canned, drained)

1 tablespoon lemon juice

1 teaspoon olive oil

Salt and pepper

Fresh dill or parsley

Mash the avocado with olive oil, lemon juice, salt, and pepper in a bowl.

Evenly top the pieces of toasted whole-grain bread with mashed avocado.

Evenly flake cooked salmon over the toast to cover the avocado.

For extra taste, top with chopped parsley or fresh dill (optional).

Egg Muffins with Spinach and Cheese

(per serving, 1 muffin):

Calories: 100

Protein: 8g

Fat: 6g

Carbs: 2g

Fiber: 1g

Calcium: 120 mg

Prep Time: 10 minutes Cooking Time: 20 minutes

6 large eggs

1/2 cup low-fat milk

1 cup fresh spinach, chopped

1/2 cup shredded cheddar cheese

1/4 teaspoon garlic powder

Salt and pepper

Olive oil or cooking spray

1/2 teaspoon ground turmeric

1/4 teaspoon ground cinnamon

1/4 teaspoon ground ginger

A handful of spinach

Set the oven's temperature to 350°F (175°C). Coat a 12-cup muffin pan with cooking spray or olive oil.

Beat the eggs, milk, salt, pepper, and garlic powder in a big basin.

Mix in the shredded cheese and the chopped spinach.

Using an even pouring motion, fill each prepared muffin tin cup approximately two thirds of the way.

Bake the egg muffins for 18 to 20 minutes, or until the tops are lightly browned and the muffins are set.

Before serving, let it cool somewhat. For a convenient grab-and-go breakfast, enjoy warm or store in the refrigerator for up to three days.

Sweet Potato Hash with Poached Eggs

(per serving, serves 2):

Calories: 300

Protein: 12g

Fat: 12g

Carbs: 36g

Fiber: 6g

Calcium: 100 mg

Prep Time: 10 minutes Cooking Time: 15 minutes

2 medium sweet potatoes, peeled and diced

1 tablespoon olive oil

1/2 onion, finely chopped

1 red bell pepper, diced

2 cloves garlic, minced

1/2 teaspoon paprika

Salt and pepper

4 large eggs

Fresh parsley

Dice the veggies and peel the sweet potatoes.

Prepare the Hash:

In a big pan over medium heat, warm up the olive oil.

Add the bell pepper, onion, and cubed sweet potatoes. Cook, stirring occasionally, until the sweet potatoes are soft and beginning to crisp, approximately 10 to 12 minutes.

Add the paprika, minced garlic, salt, and pepper. Cook the garlic for a further one to two minutes, or until fragrant.

Poach the Eggs:

Simmer a little saucepan of water and mix in a tiny amount of vinegar (optional; keeps the eggs cohesive).

One by one, crack the eggs into a small dish and carefully place them in the water that is simmering. Cook for a firmer yolk or an additional 4 minutes for soft poached eggs.

Using a slotted spoon, remove and place on paper towels to drain.

Spoon the sweet potato hash onto each dish, then place a poached egg on top of each. If desired, garnish with fresh parsley.

Eggs Benedict with a Spinach Salad

(per serving, 2 Eggs Benedict with salad):

Calories: 450

Protein: 24g

Fat: 28g

Carbs: 28g

Fiber: 4g

Calcium: 150 mg

Prep Time: 15 minutes Cooking Time: 15 minutes

For the Eggs Benedict:

2 whole wheat English muffins, split

4 large eggs

4 slices of smoked salmon or lean turkey

1 tablespoon white vinegar

For the Hollandaise Sauce:

2 egg yolks

1 tablespoon lemon juice

1/4 cup unsalted butter, melted

Pinch of salt and pepper

For the Spinach Salad:

2 cups fresh spinach

1 tablespoon olive oil

1 tablespoon balsamic vinegar

1/4 cup cherry tomatoes, halved

1/4 small red onion, thinly sliced

Eggs Benedict:

Toast the English muffins made with whole wheat and set them aside.

Pour 1 tablespoon of white vinegar into a pot, cover and bring to a boil. One by one, crack eggs into little cups and submerge them in the water. The yolks should stay liquid and the whites should solidify after 3–4 minutes of poaching. Using a slotted spoon, remove.

Whisk the egg yolks and lemon juice together in a heat-resistant dish. Slowly whisk in the melted butter while keeping the bowl over a saucepan of hot water (double boiler). Whisk the sauce continuously for approximately three minutes, or until it thickens. To taste, add salt and pepper for seasoning.

Top each half of an English muffin with a piece of turkey or smoked salmon.

Place a poached egg on top and pour hollandaise sauce over it.

Spinach Salad: Combine the red onion, cherry tomatoes, olive oil, and balsamic vinegar in a dish with the fresh spinach.

Oatmeal with Ground Flax Seeds

(per serving, 1 cup cooked oatmeal with flax seeds):

Calories: 250

Protein: 7g

Fat: 8g

Carbs: 36g

Fiber: 6g

Calcium: 300 mg

Prep Time: 5 minutes Cooking Time: 10 minutes

1 cup rolled oats

2 cups unsweetened almond milk

1 tablespoon ground flax seeds

1 tablespoon honey or maple syrup

1/2 teaspoon vanilla extract

Fresh fruit or nuts

Place the almond milk and rolled oats in a medium pot.

Over medium heat, bring to a boil, then lower the heat and simmer until the oats are soft and the mixture thickens, stirring periodically, for approximately 5 minutes.

Cook for an extra minute after stirring in the ground flax seeds.

You may add vanilla essence, honey, or maple syrup if you'd like. Mix thoroughly.

Ladle into dishes, garnish with nuts or fresh fruit, if you want.

Fortified Cereal with Milk and Banana

(per serving):

Serving Size: 1 bowl

Calories: 300

Protein: 10g

Fat: 6g

Carbs: 50g

Fiber: 7g

Calcium: 350 mg

Prep Time: 5 minutes **Cooking Time:** None

1 cup fortified whole grain cereal

1 cup low-fat milk

1 medium banana, sliced

1 tablespoon chia seeds

1 teaspoon honey or maple syrup

Cut the banana into tiny circles.

Fill a bowl with the strengthened cereal.

Douse the cereal with milk.

Top with the chia seeds, if using, and the banana slices.

If desired, drizzle maple syrup or honey over the top.

Fortified Almond Milk Smoothie with Kale

(per serving):

Serving Size: 1 smoothie (about 16 oz)

Calories: 250

Protein: 6g

Fat: 7g

Carbs: 38g

Fiber: 6g

Calcium: 450 mg

Prep Time: 5 minutes Cooking Time: None

1 cup fortified almond milk

1 cup fresh kale leaves, stems removed

1 ripe banana

1 tablespoon chia seeds

1/2 cup frozen pineapple chunks

1/2 teaspoon honey or maple syrup

Ice cubes

Peel the banana and cut the stems off of the kale leaves.

Put the frozen pineapple, kale, banana, chia seeds, almond milk, and honey (if using) in a blender. Process till smooth.

If you want a thicker texture, add ice cubes and mix until the right consistency is achieved.

Smoothie Bowl with Fortified Soy Milk

(per serving):

Serving Size: 1 bowl

Calories: 250

Protein: 8g

Fat: 6g

Carbohydrates: 38g

Fiber: 7g

Calcium: 300 mg

Prep Time: 5 minutes Cooking Time: None

1 cup fortified soy milk	Toppings:
1 cup mixed berries	1/4 cup granola
1 handful fresh spinach about 1 cup	Fresh berries
1 tablespoon chia seeds	Sliced banana
1 tablespoon honey or maple syrup	A few mint leaves
1/2 teaspoon vanilla extract	

Blend together the fortified soy milk, spinach, chia seeds (if using), honey (if using), and vanilla extract (if using) in a blender. Process till smooth.

Transfer the smoothie onto a bowl and garnish with granola, chopped mint leaves, fresh berries, and sliced banana, if preferred.

Sardines on Whole Grain Crackers

(per serving of 6 crackers with toppings):

Calories: 300

Protein: 16g

Fat: 18g

Carbs: 20g

Fiber: 4g

Calcium: 250 mg

Prep Time: 5 minutes Cooking Time: None

1 can (3.75 oz) sardines in olive oil or water, drained

6 whole grain crackers, rye or oat

1 cup fresh arugula

1 tablespoon lemon juice

1 teaspoon olive oil

Salt and pepper

Take out and reserve the sardines.

Position the whole grain crackers onto a platter for presentation.

Top each cracker with two to three sardines.

Place a few fresh arugula leaves on top of each cracker with a sardine topping.

Pour over some olive oil and lemon juice (if using). To taste, add salt and pepper for seasoning.

You may eat this right away or save it for a light snack.

Fortified Orange Juice and Whole-Grain Toast

(per serving):

Calories: 340

Protein: 6g

Fat: 20g

Carbs: 35g

Fiber: 10g

Calcium: 300 mg

Prep Time: 5 minutes Cooking Time: 3-5 minutes

1 cup fortified orange juice (calcium-fortified)

For the Whole-Grain Toast with Avocado:

2 slices whole-grain bread

1 ripe avocado

1 tablespoon lemon juice

Salt and pepper

Red pepper flakes or herbs

For the Orange Juice Fortified: Fill a glass with one cup of fortified orange juice. If store-bought fortified juice is being used, no further preparation is required.

Toast the pieces of whole-grain bread until they are as crispy as you want.

Halve the avocado, remove the pit, and scoop out the flesh into a dish while the bread is browning. Use a fork to mash, and then, if desired, stir in lemon juice.

Add salt, pepper, and extra herbs or red pepper flakes to taste while preparing the mashed avocado.

Evenly distribute the avocado mixture over the pieces of toast.

Quinoa Porridge with Almond Butter

(per serving, 1 bowl):

Calories: 270

Protein: 8g

Fat: 12g

Carbs: 36g

Fiber: 6g

Calcium: 150 mg

Prep Time: 5 minutes Cooking Time: 20 minutes

1/2 cup quinoa

1 cup water or low-fat milk

1/2 teaspoon cinnamon (optional)

1 tablespoon almond butter

1 tablespoon ground flax seeds

1 tablespoon honey or maple syrup

Fresh fruit or nuts

To get rid of any bitterness, rinse the quinoa in cold water.

Heat the milk or water in a small pot until it boils. Reduce to a simmer after adding the quinoa. After the liquid has been absorbed and the quinoa is soft, simmer it covered for approximately fifteen minutes.

Cook for an extra two minutes after stirring in the cinnamon, if using.

Take off the heat and mix in the ground flax seeds and almond butter. Blend until well blended.

You may add more sweetness by stirring in honey or maple syrup if you'd like.

Ladle the porridge into dishes, garnishing with nuts or fresh fruit, if preferred.

Buckwheat Pancakes with Walnuts

Prep Time: 10 minutes Cooking Time: 10 minutes

(per serving, 2 pancakes with toppings):

Calories: 290

Protein: 10g

Fat: 15g

Carbs: 30g

Fiber: 4g

Calcium: 150 mg

1 cup buckwheat flour

1 tablespoon baking powder

1/2 teaspoon salt

1 tablespoon honey or maple syrup

1 large egg

1 cup low-fat milk

2 tablespoons olive oil or melted butter

1/2 teaspoon vanilla extract

1/4 cup chopped walnuts

Maple syrup

Turn up the heat to medium on a nonstick skillet or griddle.

Combine the buckwheat flour, baking powder, and salt in a large basin.

Beat the egg in a separate dish, then stir in the milk, butter, honey, or syrup, and vanilla essence.

Gently swirl the dry ingredients into the wet components until they are just incorporated, being careful not to overmix.

Drizzle the griddle or pan with a little oil. For each pancake, add 1/4 cup of batter to the skillet. Cook until surface bubbles appear, then turn and continue cooking until the other side is golden brown.

Drizzle maple syrup and sprinkle chopped walnuts over pancakes..

SNACKS AND SMOOTHIES

Almonds and Dried Figs

(per serving, 1/4 cup of almonds and 1/4 cup of dried figs):

Calories: 200

Protein: 5g

Fat: 10g

Carbs: 25g

Fiber: 4g

Calcium: 120 mg

Prep Time: 5 minutes Cooking Time: None

1/2 cup raw almonds

1/2 cup dried figs (unsweetened, chopped if large)

Scoop out the dried figs and almonds.

In a dish, mix together the almonds and dried figs.

Eat as a snack right away, or refrigerate for up to a week in an airtight container.

Cheese and Whole Grain Crackers

(per serving of 4 crackers with cheese):

Calories: 220

Protein: 10g

Fat: 10g

Carbs: 22g

Fiber: 3g

Calcium: 250 mg

Prep Time: 5 minutes Cooking Time: None

4 whole grain crackers

2 ounces (about 1/4 cup) low-fat cheese LIKE cheddar, gouda, or Swiss

1/2 small apple or pear, sliced

Cut the cheese into little cubes or thin slices.

Place the cheese cubes or slices on top of the whole grain crackers.

For a cool twist, place apple or pear slices on the side.

You may eat it right away or save it for a snack.

Fortified Almond Milk Latte

(per serving, 1 cup):

Calories: 60

Protein: 1g

Fat: 3g

Carbs: 8g

Fiber: 1g

Calcium: 450 mg

Prep Time: 5 minutes Cooking Time: 5 minutes

1 cup fortified almond milk

1 shot of espresso or 1/2 cup strong brewed coffee

1 tablespoon almond butter

1/2 teaspoon vanilla extract

Sweetener of choice

Place the almond milk in a small saucepan and heat it over medium heat, without letting it boil. Blend the almond butter into the milk completely if you're using it.

Whip the heated almond milk into a creamy, frothy froth using a milk frother or whisk.

Brew a shot of espresso or 1/2 cup of strong coffee.

Fill a cup with the brewed coffee. Top with the frothed almond milk.

Add sweetener and vanilla essence, if using.

Kale Chips

(per serving, about 1 cup):

Calories: 80

Protein: 2g

Fat: 6g

Carbs: 7g

Fiber: 1g

Calcium: 150 mg

Prep Time: 10 minutes Cooking Time: 10-15 minutes

1 bunch kale, washed and dried

1 tablespoon olive oil

1/4 teaspoon sea salt

1/4 teaspoon garlic powder

1/4 teaspoon smoked paprika

Set the oven's temperature to 350°F (175°C). Use parchment paper to line a baking sheet.

Tear the kale leaves into bite-sized pieces after removing the stems.

Toss the kale pieces with olive oil in a big dish, being sure to coat them all the same. Add sea salt and any other ingredients you like, such as smoky paprika or garlic powder.

Arrange the kale pieces on the prepared baking sheet in a single layer. Bake for 10-15 minutes, or until the kale is crispy and slightly browned at the edges. To avoid burning, check often.

Before serving, take it out of the oven and let it cool.

String Cheese with Grapes

(per serving):

Calories: 160

Protein: 10g

Fat: 10g

Carbs: 12g

Fiber: 1g

Calcium: 200 mg

Prep Time: 5 minutes Cooking Time: None

1 serving of string cheese about 1 ounce

1/2 cup fresh grapes (red or green)

Thoroughly wash and pat dry the grapes.

Arrange the grapes and string cheese in a snack container or on a platter.

Sardines on Whole Wheat Crackers

(per serving, 6 crackers with sardines):

Calories: 220

Protein: 15g

Fat: 10g

Carbs: 20g

Fiber: 3g

Calcium: 400 mg

Prep Time: 5 minutes Cooking Time: None

1 can (3.75 oz) sardines in water or olive oil, drained

6 whole wheat crackers

1 tablespoon lemon juice

1 tablespoon chopped fresh parsley

1/4 teaspoon black pepper

1/4 teaspoon paprika

If the sardines are whole, split them into tiny pieces with a gentle hand.

Combine the sardines, black pepper, and lemon juice (if using) in a dish.

Top each whole wheat cracker equally with the sardine mixture.

If preferred, top with finely chopped parsley.

Pineapple-Ginger Smoothie

(per serving, about 1 1/2 cups):

Prep Time: 5 minutes Cooking Time: None

Calories: 210

Protein: 10g

Fat: 5g

Carbs: 30g

Fiber: 5g

Calcium: 300 mg

1 cup fresh pineapple chunks or canned in its own juice, drained

1/2 cup low-fat Greek yogurt

1/2 cup unsweetened almond milk (calcium-fortified) or any non-dairy milk

1 teaspoon fresh ginger, grated

1 tablespoon chia seeds

1 teaspoon honey or maple syrup

Ice cubes

Chop the fresh pineapple into bits if using it. Finely chop the newly harvested ginger.

Grated ginger, pineapple, Greek yogurt, almond milk, and chia seeds (if used) should all be combined in a blender. If preferred, add maple syrup or honey. Process till smooth.

Blend again after adding a few ice cubes if you'd like your smoothie thicker.

Kale and Banana Smoothie

(per serving):

Serving Size: 1 smoothie (about 12 oz)

Calories: 220

Protein: 12g

Fat: 5g

Carbs: 32g

Fiber: 6g

Calcium: 300 mg

Prep Time: 5 minutes Cooking Time: None

1 cup fresh kale leaves, stems removed

1 ripe banana

1/2 cup plain Greek yogurt

1/2 cup unsweetened almond milk

1 tablespoon chia seeds

1 teaspoon honey or maple syrup

1/2 cup ice

Remove the stems and give the kale a good wash. Grab the banana and peel it.

Put the kale, banana, almond milk, Greek yogurt, and chia seeds (if using) in a blender. Add honey or syrup if preferred for sweetness.

Purée until well combined. Add ice and process the smoothie once more if you'd like it cooler.

Mixed Berry and Spinach Smoothie

(per serving):

Serving Size: 1 smoothie (about 12 ounces)

Calories: 250

Protein: 10g

Fat: 6g

Carbs: 36g

Fiber: 7g

Calcium: 300 mg

Prep Time: 5 minutes Cooking Time: None

1 cup fresh spinach leaves

1 cup mixed berries

1 banana

1/2 cup plain Greek yogurt (calcium-fortified)

1/2 cup unsweetened almond milk

1 tablespoon chia seeds

1 teaspoon honey or maple syrup

Ice cubes

Fill a blender with all the ingredients.

Blend until smooth on high. If you like a thicker texture, feel free to add ice cubes.

Mango and Orange Smoothie

(per serving):

Serving Size: 1 glass (about 1 1/2 cups)

Calories: 250

Protein: 8g

Fat: 5g

Carbs: 35g

Fiber: 5g

Calcium: 300 mg

Prep Time: 5 minutes Cooking Time: None

1 cup fresh or frozen mango chunks

1/2 cup fresh orange juice (preferably 100% pure)

1/2 cup low-fat Greek yogurt

1/2 cup unsweetened almond milk or other calcium-fortified non-dairy milk

1 tablespoon chia seeds

1 teaspoon honey or maple syrup

Put the mango chunks, almond milk, Greek yogurt, orange juice, and chia seeds (if using) in a blender.

If you would like your smoothie to be sweeter, add honey or maple syrup.

Purée until velvety and silky.

MEAT, SEAFOOD, FISH AND PROTEIN

Grilled Chicken with Spinach

(per serving, including 1 grilled chicken breast and 1 cup salad):

Calories: 350

Protein: 30g

Fat: 15g

Carbs: 25g

Fiber: 4g

Calcium: 150 mg

Prep Time: 15 minutes Cooking Time: 20 minutes

For the Grilled Chicken:

2 boneless, skinless chicken breasts

1 tablespoon olive oil

1 teaspoon garlic powder

1 teaspoon paprika

Salt and black pepper

1 tablespoon lemon juice

For the Spinach and Quinoa Salad:

1 cup quinoa

2 cups water

4 cups fresh spinach leaves

1/2 cup cherry tomatoes, halved

1/4 cup sliced red onion

1/4 cup crumbled feta cheese

2 tablespoons olive oil

1 tablespoon balsamic vinegar

Salt and black pepper

For the Grilled Chicken:

Combine the olive oil, paprika, garlic powder, salt, pepper, and lemon juice in a small bowl. The chicken breasts should be rubbed with the mixture and let marinade for at least half an hour.

Turn the heat up to medium-high. The chicken should be cooked through after grilling for 6–7 minutes on each side, or until the internal temperature reaches 165°F/74°C. Take off of the grill and let it a five-minute rest before slicing.

Regarding the Quinoa and Spinach Salad:

Wash the quinoa in cool water. Bring two cups of water to a boil in a medium saucepan. After adding the quinoa, lower the heat, cover, and simmer until the water is absorbed—about 15 minutes. Using a fork, fluff and let to cool.

The cooked quinoa, spinach, cherry tomatoes, red onion, and feta cheese (if using) should all be combined in a big bowl.

Combine the olive oil, balsamic vinegar, salt, and pepper in a small bowl. Drizzle the salad with the dressing and mix well.

Turkey Chili with Beans

(per serving, about 1 cup):

Calories: 280

Protein: 20g

Fat: 8g

Carbs: 30g

Fiber: 8g

Calcium: 150 mg

Prep Time: 15 minutes Cooking Time: 30 minutes

1 lb ground turkey (lean)

1 tablespoon olive oil

1 onion, diced

2 cloves garlic, minced

1 bell pepper, diced

1 can (14.5 oz) diced tomatoes

1 can (15 oz) kidney beans, drained and rinsed

1 can (15 oz) black beans, drained and rinsed

1 cup low-sodium chicken broth

2 tablespoons chili powder

1 teaspoon cumin

1/2 teaspoon paprika

1/2 teaspoon oregano

Salt and pepper

Optional Toppings:

1/2 cup shredded low-fat cheddar cheese

Fresh cilantro, chopped

Sliced avocado

Heat the olive oil in a large saucepan over medium heat. Using a spoon, break up the ground turkey while it cooks until it becomes brown. When necessary, drain extra fat.

Include the bell pepper, onion, and garlic in the saucepan. Cook for approximately 5 minutes, or until the veggies are tender.

Add the oregano, cumin, paprika, chili powder, black beans, kidney beans, and chopped tomatoes. Heat till boiling.

Lower the heat and simmer the chili for twenty to twenty-five minutes, or until the chili has thickened and the flavors are thoroughly blended. To taste, add salt and pepper for seasoning.

Spoon chili into bowls; garnish with avocado, shredded cheese, and cilantro, if using.

Lamb Chops with Kale and Sweet Potatoes

(per serving):

Serving Size: 1 lamb chop with 1/4 of the sweet potatoes and kale

Calories: 350

Protein: 26g

Fat: 22g

Carbs: 25g

Fiber: 5g

Calcium: 150 mg

Prep Time: 15 minutes Cooking Time: 30 minutes

4 lamb chops (about 1 inch thick)

2 tablespoons olive oil

1 teaspoon dried rosemary

1 teaspoon dried thyme

Salt and black pepper to taste

2 medium sweet potatoes, peeled and cut into 1-inch cubes

4 cups kale, stems removed and chopped

3 cloves garlic, minced

1 tablespoon lemon juice

1/4 cup water or low-sodium broth

Set oven temperature to 400°F, or 200°C. Add one tablespoon of olive oil, salt, and pepper to the sweet potato cubes and toss. Transfer them onto a baking sheet and bake for 25 to 30 minutes, or until they become soft and start to turn golden brown.

Sprinkle the lamb chops with salt, pepper, rosemary, and thyme while the sweet potatoes roast. In a large pan, heat the remaining olive oil over medium-high heat. After adding the lamb chops, grill them for 4–5 minutes on each side, or until they are cooked to your liking. Take out of the skillet and let it sit aside to rest.

Add the minced garlic to the same pan and sauté for about one minute, or until fragrant. Add the water (or broth) and chopped greens. Cook the kale for 5 to 7 minutes, stirring regularly, or until it is soft and wilted. Add the lemon juice and season to taste with salt and pepper.

Arrange the sautéed kale and roasted sweet potatoes on a platter with the lamb chops.

Baked Chicken Thighs with Garlic

(per serving, 1 chicken thigh with spinach):

Calories: 280

Protein: 23g

Fat: 18g

Carbs: 4g

Fiber: 1g

Calcium: 60 mg

Prep Time: 10 minutes Cooking Time: 35 minutes

4 bone-in, skinless chicken thighs

2 tablespoons olive oil

4 cloves garlic, minced

1 cup fresh spinach leaves

1 teaspoon dried oregano

1 teaspoon dried thyme

1/2 teaspoon paprika

Salt and pepper

1/2 lemon, juiced

Set the oven temperature to 400°F, or 200°C.

Use paper towels to pat the chicken thighs dry. Garlic, oregano, thyme, paprika, olive oil, salt, and pepper should be rubbed on them.

Transfer the chicken thighs to a baking dish or a sheet covered with parchment paper. Bake the chicken for 30 to 35 minutes, or until the skin is crispy and the internal temperature reaches 165°F (74°C).

Arrange the spinach leaves around the chicken on the baking pan about ten minutes before the chicken is done. Bake the spinach until it begins to wilt.

Before serving, you might choose to drizzle some lemon juice over the chicken.

Sardines on Whole-Grain Toast

(per serving, 1 slice of toast with sardines):

Calories: 250

Protein: 15g

Fat: 12g

Carbs: 22g

Fiber: 4g

Calcium: 250 mg

Prep Time: 5 minutes Cooking Time: 3 minutes

1 can (3.75 oz) sardines in water or olive oil, drained

2 slices whole-grain bread

1 tablespoon olive oil (if using sardines in water)

1 tablespoon lemon juice

1 tablespoon chopped fresh parsley or basil

1/4 teaspoon black pepper

1/4 teaspoon garlic powder

1/4 teaspoon red pepper flakes

Use a toaster or toaster oven to toast the whole-grain bread pieces until they are golden brown.

In a pan over medium heat, warm the olive oil if using sardines in water. Sardines should be added and cooked for two to three minutes to fully reheat. For sardines cooked in oil, omit this step.

Combine the sardines, lemon juice, garlic powder, parsley or basil, black pepper, and red pepper flakes (if using) in a dish.

Evenly distribute the sardine mixture over the pieces of toasted whole-grain bread.

Savor the dish right away, and if you'd like, top with more parsley or basil.

Mackerel with Olive Oil and Roasted Vegetables

Prep Time: 15 minutes Cooking Time: 30 minutes

(per serving, 1 mackerel filet with vegetables):

Calories**: 370

Protein: 30g

Fat: 22g

Carbs: 22g

Fiber: 5g

Calcium: 150 mg

2 mackerel filets about 6 oz each

2 tablespoons olive oil

1 lemon, sliced

1 teaspoon dried thyme or fresh if available

1/2 teaspoon garlic powder

Salt and pepper

For Roasted Vegetables:

1 medium sweet potato, peeled and diced

1 bell pepper, chopped

1 zucchini, sliced

1 red onion, chopped

1 tablespoon olive oil

1/2 teaspoon dried rosemary

Salt and pepper

Set the oven's temperature to 400°F, or 200°C.

Combine olive oil, rosemary, salt, and pepper with the sweet potato, bell pepper, zucchini, and red onion. Arrange them on a baking sheet in a single layer.

Roast for 20 to 25 minutes, or until soft and beginning to caramelize, in a preheated oven.

Make the mackerel while the veggies are roasting. Put the filets on an ovenproof dish or separate baking sheet. Season with salt, pepper, dried thyme, and garlic powder. Drizzle with olive oil. Add slices of lemon on top.

During the last ten minutes of the vegetable roasting process, place the mackerel in the oven (on a different rack). Once the mackerel is cooked through and flakes easily with a fork, bake it for ten minutes.

Present the mackerel right away by plating it with roasted vegetables.

Shrimp Stir-Fry with Bok Choy

(per serving, based on 4 servings):

Calories: 250

Protein: 22g

Fat: 10g

Carbs: 18g

Fiber: 4g

Calcium: 150 mg

Prep Time: 10 minutes Cooking Time: 10 minutes

1 lb (450g) large shrimp, peeled and deveined

1 tablespoon olive oil

2 cloves garlic, minced

1 tablespoon fresh ginger, minced

2 cups bok choy, chopped (both stems and leaves)

1 red bell pepper, sliced

1 cup snap peas or green beans

2 tablespoons low-sodium soy sauce or tamari

1 tablespoon rice vinegar

1 teaspoon sesame oil

1 tablespoon sesame seeds

Cooked brown rice or quinoa

Cut up veggies and get ready to make shrimp.

In a large pan or wok, heat the olive oil over medium-high heat. Add the ginger and garlic and simmer for approximately a minute, or until fragrant. Add the shrimp and simmer for 3–4 minutes, or until they are pink and opaque. Take out of the pan and place the shrimp aside.

Place snap peas, bell pepper, and bok choy in the same pan. Stir-fry the veggies for 4–5 minutes, or until they are crisp-tender.

Transfer the shrimp back to the skillet. Stir in sesame oil, rice vinegar, and soy sauce. After thoroughly mixing, cook for a further two minutes.

If preferred, garnish with sesame seeds. Serve with cooked quinoa or brown rice.

Baked Trout with Lemon and Garlic

(per serving, 1 filet):

Calories: 220

Protein: 22g

Fat: 12g

Carbs: 2g

Fiber: 1g

Calcium: 50 mg

Prep Time: 10 minutes Cooking Time: 15-20 minutes

2 trout filets about 6 oz each

2 tablespoons olive oil

2 cloves garlic, minced

1 lemon, thinly sliced

1 tablespoon fresh parsley, chopped (optional)

Salt and pepper

Lemon wedges

Set the oven's temperature to 375°F, or 190°C.

Arrange the fish filets on a baking sheet that has been gently oiled or coated with parchment paper.

Toss in the minced garlic and drizzle with olive oil over the filets. To taste, add salt and pepper for seasoning.

Top the filets with slices of lemon.

Bake the fish for 15 to 20 minutes, or until a fork can easily pierce it.

If wanted, garnish with fresh parsley and serve with slices of lemon.

Tuna Salad with Spinach and Avocado

(per serving, about 1 1/2 cups):

Prep Time: 10 minutes Cooking Time: None

Calories: 320

Protein: 23g

Fat: 20g

Carbs: 14g

Fiber: 8g

Calcium: 150 mg

1 can (5 oz) tuna in water, drained

1 cup fresh spinach leaves, chopped

1 ripe avocado, diced

1/4 cup red onion, finely chopped

1/4 cup cherry tomatoes, halved

1 tablespoon olive oil

1 tablespoon lemon juice

Salt and pepper

1 tablespoon chopped fresh parsley

Combine the diced avocado, cherry tomatoes, red onion, and spinach in a big bowl.

Fill the bowl with the drained tuna.

Squeeze in some lemon juice and olive oil. To taste, add salt and pepper for seasoning.

Gently toss everything until well mixed.

If wanted, garnish with fresh parsley and serve right away.

Cod with Tomato and Olive Relish

(per serving, 1 cod filet with relish):

Calories: 250

Protein: 25g

Fat: 14g

Carbs: 10g

Fiber: 3g

Calcium: 80 mg

Prep Time: 15 minutes Cooking Time: 15 minutes

For the Cod:

4 cod filets (about 6 oz each)

2 tablespoons olive oil

Salt and pepper

1 lemon, sliced

For the Tomato and Olive Relish:

1 cup cherry tomatoes, halved

1/2 cup black olives, pitted and sliced

1/4 cup red onion, finely chopped

2 tablespoons capers, rinsed

2 tablespoons olive oil

1 tablespoon balsamic vinegar

2 cloves garlic, minced

1 tablespoon fresh basil or parsley, chopped

Salt and pepper

Set the oven's temperature to 400°F, or 200°C.

Arrange the fish filets on a parchment paper-lined baking sheet. Add a drizzle of olive oil and season with pepper and salt. Arrange slices of lemon over the filets.

Bake the fish for 12 to 15 minutes, or until it is opaque and flakes readily with a fork, in a preheated oven.

As the fish bakes, make the relish

In a bowl, mix together cherry tomatoes, black olives, red onion, capers, olive oil, balsamic vinegar, garlic, and fresh basil (or parsley). Stir well and add pepper and salt to taste.

Take the cod out of the oven and place it on serving platters. Serve the fish right away after spooning the tomato and olive relish on top of it.

Herring with Beet and Arugula Salad

Prep Time: 10 minutes Cooking Time: 30 minutes

(per serving, 1/4 of salad with herring):

Calories: 250

Protein: 15g

Fat: 16g

Carbs: 15g

Fiber: 4g

Calcium: 200 mg

For the Salad:

2 medium beets, peeled and diced

2 cups fresh arugula

1/4 cup crumbled goat cheese

1/4 cup chopped walnuts

1 tablespoon olive oil

1 tablespoon balsamic vinegar

Salt and pepper

For the Herring:

4 oz pickled herring filets, drained or fresh herring, grilled or baked

1 tablespoon chopped fresh dill or 1 teaspoon dried dill

Lemon wedges for serving

Set oven temperature to 400°F, or 200°C. On a baking sheet, spread some olive oil over the diced beets, then season with salt and pepper. Roast until soft, 25 to 30 minutes. Let it cool.

Combine the fresh arugula and roasted beets in a large dish. If using, add the walnuts and goat cheese.

Drizzle with balsamic vinegar and olive oil. Gently toss to mix.

To assemble pickled herring on a platter, cut it into small pieces using a knife. If you are using fresh herring, season with dill and bake or grill until done. Accompany with slices of lemon.

Transfer salad to plates, then sprinkle herring on top. Serve right away.

Lentil Stew with Carrots and Spinach

(per serving, 1 cup):

Calories: 180

Protein: 10g

Fat: 4g

Carbs: 30g

Fiber: 8g

Calcium: 90 mg

Prep Time: 10 minutes Cooking Time: 35-40 minutes

1 tablespoon olive oil

1 medium onion, chopped

2 garlic cloves, minced

2 medium carrots, diced

1 cup dried green or brown lentils, rinsed

1 can (14.5 oz) diced tomatoes

4 cups vegetable broth

2 cups fresh spinach, chopped

1 teaspoon ground cumin

1/2 teaspoon ground turmeric

1/2 teaspoon paprika

Salt and pepper

In a large saucepan over medium heat, warm the olive oil. Add the onion and garlic, and simmer for approximately 5 minutes, or until softened.

Cook for a further five minutes after stirring in the carrots.

Stir in the paprika, cumin, turmeric, lentils, chopped tomatoes, vegetable broth, salt, and pepper. Heat till boiling.

Lower the heat and simmer the lentils for 25 to 30 minutes, covered, or until they become soft.

Add the spinach, stir, and simmer until wilted, about 5 more minutes.

Serve hot, adjusting the spice as necessary.

Black Bean and Sweet Potato Enchiladas

(per serving, 1 enchilada):

Calories: 250

Protein: 10g

Fat: 8g

Carbs: 35g

Fiber: 7g

Calcium: 150 mg

Prep Time: 15 minutes Cooking Time: 40 minutes

2 medium sweet potatoes, peeled and diced

1 tablespoon olive oil

1/2 teaspoon ground cumin

1/2 teaspoon paprika

1/2 teaspoon garlic powder

1 can (15 oz) black beans, drained and rinsed

1 cup corn kernels (fresh or frozen)

1/2 cup diced red onion

1 cup shredded cheddar cheese

8 whole wheat or corn tortillas

1 1/2 cups enchilada sauce

1/4 cup chopped fresh cilantro

Set the oven to 400°F, or 200°C. Mix the chopped sweet potatoes with paprika, garlic powder, cumin, and olive oil. Arrange on a baking sheet in a single layer.

Bake the sweet potatoes for 25 to 30 minutes, or until they are soft and starting to caramelize. Take out and put aside.

Gather the roasted sweet potatoes, black beans, corn, and finely chopped red onion in a large dish.

Lightly coat the bottom of a baking dish with enchilada sauce. Spoon the sweet potato mixture over each tortilla, fold it up, and put it seam-side down in the baking dish.

Cover the rolled tortillas with the leftover enchilada sauce. Add some cheese shreds on top.

Bake for 20 minutes in a preheated oven, covered with foil. After removing the foil, bake for a further ten minutes, or until the cheese is bubbling and melted.

Before serving, let it cool somewhat. If desired, garnish with finely chopped cilantro.

Frittata with Spinach and Mushrooms

Prep Time: 15 minutes Cooking Time: 30 minutes

(per serving, assuming 6 servings):

Calories: 180

Protein: 12g

Fat: 12g

Carbs: 5g

Fiber: 1g

Calcium: 150 mg

6 large eggs	1 tablespoon olive oil
1/2 cup milk	1/2 small onion, diced
1 cup fresh spinach, chopped	2 cloves garlic, minced
1/2 cup mushrooms, sliced	Salt and pepper
1/2 cup shredded cheese	

Set the oven's temperature to 375°F (190°C). Use a little olive oil to lightly grease a 9-inch pie plate or oven-safe pan.

Heat olive oil in a pan over a medium flame. Cook the chopped onion until it becomes transparent. Add the chopped garlic and sauté the sliced mushrooms until they become soft. Add chopped spinach and stir until it wilts. Take off the heat.

Beat eggs, milk, pepper, and salt in a bowl.

Stir to blend the cooked veggies into the egg mixture. Add the cheese as well, if using.

Transfer the mixture to the dish that has been ready. Bake for 25 to 30 minutes in a preheated oven, or until the frittata is set and has a softly brown crust.

Before slicing, let cool somewhat. Savor hot or room temperature.

VEGETARIAN AND VEGAN

Whole Wheat Pita with Hummus and Cucumber

(per serving, 1 pita with hummus and cucumber):

Calories: 220

Protein: 8g

Fat: 8g

Carbs: 28g

Fiber: 6g

Calcium: 90 mg

Prep Time: 5 minutes Cooking Time: None

1 whole wheat pita bread

1/4 cup hummus (store-bought or homemade)

1/2 cucumber, sliced

1 tablespoon chopped fresh parsley

1/2 teaspoon lemon juice

Salt and pepper

You may either leave the whole wheat pita bread whole or cut it in half to make pockets.

If you are not cutting into the pita pockets, evenly distribute the hummus within them or on top of them.

Place sliced cucumber over the hummus.

If preferred, top with chopped parsley, lemon juice, salt, and pepper.

If making ahead, chill or eat right away.

Cheesy Broccoli and Mushroom Omelette

Prep Time: 10 minutes Cooking Time: 10 minutes

(per serving):

Calories: 270

Protein: 18g

Fat: 19g

Carbs: 8g

Fiber: 3g

Calcium: 300 mg

2 large eggs	Salt and pepper to taste
1/4 cup low-fat shredded cheese	1/4 teaspoon garlic powder
1/2 cup broccoli florets, chopped	1/4 teaspoon onion powder
1/2 cup mushrooms, sliced	
1 tablespoon olive oil or cooking spray	

Cut the mushrooms into slices and chop the broccoli. Heat up a non-stick skillet to medium temperature and drizzle with olive oil or cooking spray.

Include the broccoli and mushrooms in the pan. Cook for approximately 5 minutes, stirring periodically, or until the broccoli is soft and the mushrooms are golden brown. If desired, add onion, garlic, and salt powder for seasoning.

Beat the eggs in a basin while the veggies are boiling. Add a dash of pepper and salt for seasoning.

Cover the sautéed veggies in the pan with the beaten eggs. After letting the eggs set around the edges, carefully remove them with a spatula to allow any remaining egg to slide below. Over one side of the omelet, equally distribute the shredded cheese.

Fold the omelet in half over the cheese after the tops of the eggs are largely set but still somewhat runny. Cook the omelet for a further one to two minutes, or until the cheese has melted and it is well cooked.

Transfer the omelet to a platter and start eating right away.

Whole-Grain Pasta with Pesto and Parmesan

Prep Time: 10 minutes Cooking Time: 10 minutes

(per serving, 1 cup pasta with pesto and Parmesan):

Calories: 320

Protein: 12g

Fat: 14g

Carbs: 36g

Fiber: 5g

Calcium: 250 mg

8 ounces whole-grain pasta

1/2 cup homemade or store-bought pesto (preferably with added nuts like pine nuts or almonds for extra calcium)

1/4 cup grated Parmesan cheese

1 tablespoon olive oil

1/4 cup chopped pine nuts

Salt and pepper

Fill a big pot with boiling salted water. When the pasta is al dente, add the whole-grain variety and boil it as directed on the box. Empty and put back into the pot.

Stir in the pesto until it coats the pasta evenly while it's still warm. Stir in the olive oil after adding it.

Drizzle the spaghetti with the grated Parmesan cheese and mix well.

Add chopped pine nuts to the mixture for added calcium and crunch.

Sprinkle it with pepper and salt to taste, and serve right away.

Tofu Scramble with Spinach

(per serving, about 1 cup):

Prep Time: 10 minutes Cooking Time: 15 minutes

Calories: 200

Protein: 15g

Fat: 12g

Carbs: 12g

Fiber: 4g

Calcium: 300 mg

1 block (14 oz) firm tofu, drained and crumbled

1 tablespoon olive oil

1 small onion, diced

1 red bell pepper, diced

1 green bell pepper, diced

2 cups fresh spinach, chopped

1/2 teaspoon turmeric powder

1/2 teaspoon garlic powder

1/2 teaspoon onion powder

Salt and black pepper

1 tablespoon nutritional yeast

Using your hands or a fork, crumble the tofu into tiny pieces.

In a large pan set over medium heat, warm up the olive oil. Add the bell peppers and onion, chopped. When the veggies are soft, sauté them for five to seven minutes.

Fill the skillet with the smashed tofu. Add the onion, garlic, and turmeric powders along with the salt and pepper. Cook, stirring periodically, for 5 minutes

Fill the pan with the chopped spinach. Cook the spinach for a further two to three minutes, or until it wilts.

Add the nutritional yeast and mix if using. Taste and adjust seasoning.

Vegan Sweet Potato and Black Bean Tacos

(per serving, 2 tacos):

Calories: 350

Protein: 12g

Fat: 12g

Carbs: 50g

Fiber: 12g

Calcium: 100 mg

Prep Time: 10 minutes Cooking Time: 25 minutes

1 large sweet potato, peeled and diced

1 tablespoon olive oil

1/2 teaspoon smoked paprika

1/2 teaspoon ground cumin

1/2 teaspoon garlic powder

Salt and pepper to taste

1 can (15 oz) black beans, drained and rinsed

1/2 cup diced red bell pepper

1/4 cup chopped fresh cilantro

8 small corn tortillas

1 avocado, sliced

1 lime, cut into wedges

Salsa

Set the oven's temperature to 400°F (200°C). Add the smoked paprika, cumin, garlic powder, olive oil, salt, and pepper to the chopped sweet potato. Organize evenly on a baking sheet.

Roast, tossing halfway through, in a preheated oven for 20 to 25 minutes, or until soft and beginning to caramelize.

In a pan over medium heat, reheat the black beans and red bell pepper while the sweet potatoes are roasting.

Preheat the corn tortillas in an oven or dry skillet. Place roasted sweet potatoes, black beans, and bell pepper into each tortilla.

Garnish with chopped cilantro, avocado slices, and lime juice. If desired, top with more toppings or salsa.

Vegan Lentil Soup with Spinach and Carrots

(per serving, 1 cup):

Calories: 180

Protein: 10g

Fat: 5g

Carbs: 26g

Fiber: 8g

Calcium: 90 mg

Prep Time: 10 minutes Cooking Time: 40 minutes

1 tablespoon olive oil

1 large onion, diced

3 garlic cloves, minced

2 large carrots, peeled and diced

1 celery stalk, diced

1 cup dried green or brown lentils, rinsed

1 can (14.5 oz) diced tomatoes

4 cups vegetable broth

2 cups fresh spinach, chopped

1 teaspoon ground cumin

1/2 teaspoon smoked paprika

Salt and pepper

1 bay leaf (optional)

1 tablespoon lemon juice

In a large saucepan over medium heat, warm the olive oil.

Add the garlic and onion and simmer for approximately 5 minutes, or until softened. After adding the celery and carrots, simmer for a further five minutes.

Add the bay leaf (if using), cumin, smoky paprika, chopped tomatoes, and vegetable broth. Heat till boiling.

Lower the temperature to a simmer, cover the pot, and cook the soup until the lentils are soft, approximately 30 minutes.

Add the fresh spinach and simmer, stirring, until wilted, about 5 more minutes.

Season to taste with salt, pepper, and lemon juice (if using).

Fortified Soy Yogurt with Fresh Berries

(per serving):

Prep Time: 5 minutes Cooking Time: None

Serving Size: 1 cup

Calories: 220

Protein: 8g

1 cup fortified soy yogurt

Fat: 7g

1/2 cup fresh mixed berries

Carbs: 30g

1 tablespoon ground flaxseeds

Fiber: 6g

1 teaspoon honey or maple syrup

Calcium: 300 mg

Rinse and pat dry the fresh strawberries.

Place the ground flaxseeds and the fortified soy yogurt in a bowl. Mix well by stirring.

Cover the yogurt mixture with the fresh berries.

If preferred, drizzle with maple syrup or honey.

Eat right away or store in the fridge until you're ready.

Vegan Whole Grain Toast with Avocado

Prep Time: 5 minutes Cooking Time: 5 minutes

(per serving, 1 slice of toast with toppings):

Calories: 220

Protein: 6g

Fat: 14g

Carbs: 22g

Fiber: 8g

Calcium: 90 mg

2 slices whole grain bread

1 ripe avocado

1 tablespoon sesame seeds

1 tablespoon lemon juice

Salt and pepper

1/4 teaspoon red pepper flakes

Toast the pieces of whole grain bread until they are the crispiness you want.

Cut the avocado in half, remove the pit, and scoop out the flesh into a dish while the bread is browning. Using a fork, mash the avocado and season with salt, pepper, and lemon juice.

Over the toasty bread pieces, equally distribute the mashed avocado.

Top the toast with avocado and garnish with sesame seeds and red pepper flakes, if desired.

To have the greatest texture, eat right away.

Chickpea and Kale Stir-Fry with Brown Rice

Prep Time: 10 minutes Cooking Time: 20 minutes)

(per serving, 1 cup stir-fry with 1/2 cup rice):

Calories: 350

Protein: 12g

Fat: 10g

Carbs: 50g

Fiber: 10g

Calcium: 150 mg

1 cup brown rice

1 tablespoon olive oil

1 medium onion, diced

2 cloves garlic, minced

1 bell pepper, sliced

1 cup cooked chickpeas (canned, drained, or cooked from dried)

2 cups kale, chopped

1 medium carrot, sliced

2 tablespoons soy sauce or tamari for gluten-free

1 tablespoon lemon juice

1/2 teaspoon ground cumin

1/2 teaspoon smoked paprika

Salt and pepper

1 tablespoon sesame seeds

Use cold water to rinse the brown rice. After bringing two cups of water to a boil in a medium-sized saucepan, add the rice, lower the heat, cover, and simmer until the rice is cooked, 45 to 50 minutes. Using a fork, fluff and keep warm.

In a large pan or wok, heat the olive oil over medium heat while the rice is cooking. Sauté the onion and garlic for three minutes, or until they are tender.

Cook the carrot and bell pepper in the pan for a further five minutes, or until they begin to soften.

Mix in the soy sauce, cumin, smoked paprika, and chickpeas. Cook for approximately 5 minutes, stirring regularly, or until the chickpeas are cooked through and the kale has wilted.

Add salt, pepper, and lemon juice to taste. When serving, top with brown rice and, if desired, sesame seeds.

GRAINS AND LEGUMES

Quinoa Salad with Spinach, Chickpeas, and Feta

(per serving, 1 cup):

Calories: 250

Protein: 9g

Fat: 14g

Carbs: 27g

Fiber: 5g

Calcium: 150 mg

Prep Time: 15 minutes Cooking Time: 15 minutes

1 cup quinoa

2 cups water or low-sodium vegetable broth

1 cup fresh spinach leaves, chopped

1 cup canned chickpeas, drained and rinsed

1/2 cup crumbled feta cheese

1/4 cup red onion, finely chopped

1/4 cup fresh parsley, chopped

1/4 cup extra virgin olive oil

2 tablespoons lemon juice

Salt and pepper

Give it a quick rinse in cool water. Bring the vegetable broth or water to a boil in a medium-sized saucepan. After adding the quinoa, turn down the heat to low, cover, and simmer until the liquid is absorbed and the quinoa is tender—about 15 minutes. Using a fork, fluff and let to cool.

Put cooked quinoa, chopped spinach, chickpeas, feta cheese, red onion, and parsley in a big bowl.

Mix the olive oil, lemon juice, salt, and pepper in a small bowl. Drizzle the salad with the dressing and mix well.

You may eat right now or store in the fridge for later.

Lentil Soup with Kale and Carrots

(per serving, 1 cup):

Calories: 180

Protein: 10g

Fat: 5g

Carbs: 25g

Fiber: 8g

Calcium: 150 mg

Prep Time: 15 minutes Cooking Time: 40 minutes

1 tablespoon olive oil

1 onion, diced

2 garlic cloves, minced

2 carrots, peeled and diced

1 cup dried green or brown lentils, rinsed

1 can (14.5 oz) diced tomatoes (no salt added)

4 cups low-sodium vegetable broth

2 cups kale, chopped (stems removed)

1 teaspoon ground cumin

1/2 teaspoon paprika

1/2 teaspoon turmeric

Salt and pepper

1 tablespoon lemon juice

In a large saucepan over medium heat, heat the olive oil. Add the onion and garlic, and simmer for approximately 5 minutes, or until softened.

Cook for a further three minutes after stirring in the carrots.

Stir in the lentils, paprika, cumin, chopped tomatoes, and turmeric (if using). Heat till boiling.

Lower the heat to a simmer, cover, and cook until the carrots and lentils are soft, approximately 30 minutes.

Cook for a further five minutes, or until the kale has wilted, after stirring in the chopped kale.

If desired, add more salt, pepper, and lemon juice to the seasoning

Brown Rice and Black Bean

(per serving):

Serving Size: 1 bowl

Calories: 350

Protein: 12g

Fat: 15g

Carbs: 45g

Fiber: 12g

Calcium: 90 mg

Prep Time: 10 minutes Cooking Time: 45 minutes for rice + 7 minutes for beans

1 cup brown rice

1 1/2 cups water

1 can (15 oz) black beans, drained and rinsed

1 tablespoon olive oil

1 teaspoon ground cumin

1/2 teaspoon paprika

1/4 teaspoon garlic powder

Salt and pepper

1 ripe avocado, sliced

1/2 cup diced tomatoes

1/4 cup chopped fresh cilantro (optional)

1 lime, cut into wedges

Place 1 1/2 cups of water in a medium saucepan and bring to a boil. When the rice is soft and the water has been absorbed, add the brown rice, lower the heat to low, cover, and simmer for 45 minutes. Using a fork, fluff.

In a pan over medium heat, warm the olive oil while the rice cooks. Incorporate the cumin, paprika, garlic powder, black beans, salt, and pepper. Simmer for about 5 to 7 minutes, stirring often, or until well cooked and seasoned.

Spoon the cooked brown rice into individual bowls. Add chopped tomatoes, avocado slices, black beans, and, if desired, fresh cilantro on top.

Just before serving, squeeze some lime juice over the top.

Farro Salad with Roasted Vegetables

(per serving):

Serving Size: 1 bowl

Calories: 350

Protein: 12g

Fat: 15g

Carbs: 45g

Fiber: 12g

Calcium: 90 mg

Prep Time: 10 minutes Cooking Time: 45 minutes for rice + 7 minutes for beans

1 cup brown rice

1 1/2 cups water

1 can (15 oz) black beans, drained and rinsed

1 tablespoon olive oil

1 teaspoon ground cumin

1/2 teaspoon paprika

1/4 teaspoon garlic powder

Salt and pepper

1 ripe avocado, sliced

1/2 cup diced tomatoes

1/4 cup chopped fresh cilantro

1 lime, cut into wedges

Place 1 1/2 cups of water in a medium saucepan and bring to a boil. When the rice is soft and the water has been absorbed, add the brown rice, lower the heat to low, cover, and simmer for 45 minutes. Using a fork, fluff.

In a pan over medium heat, warm the olive oil while the rice cooks. Incorporate the cumin, paprika, garlic powder, black beans, salt, and pepper. Simmer for about 5 to 7 minutes, stirring often, or until well cooked and seasoned.

Spoon the cooked brown rice into individual bowls. Add chopped tomatoes, avocado slices, black beans, and, if desired, fresh cilantro on top.

Just before serving, squeeze some lime juice over the top.

Chickpea and Sweet Potato Stew

(per serving, about 1 1/2 cups):

Calories: 280

Protein: 9g

Fat: 8g

Carbs: 45g

Fiber: 10g

Calcium: 120 mg

Prep Time: 15 minutes Cooking Time: 30 minutes

1 tablespoon olive oil

1 medium onion, chopped

2 garlic cloves, minced

1 tablespoon ginger, minced

1 medium sweet potato, peeled and diced

1 can (15 oz) chickpeas, drained and rinsed

1 can (14.5 oz) diced tomatoes

1 cup vegetable broth (low-sodium)

1 teaspoon ground cumin

1 teaspoon paprika

1/2 teaspoon turmeric

1/2 teaspoon ground coriander

1/2 teaspoon ground black pepper

1/4 teaspoon salt or to taste

2 cups fresh spinach or kale, chopped

1 tablespoon fresh lemon juice

Dice the sweet potato, mince the garlic, and chop the onion.

In a large saucepan over medium heat, heat the olive oil. Add the onion and simmer for approximately 5 minutes, or until transparent. After adding the ginger and garlic, simmer for an additional minute.

Place the chopped sweet potato in the saucepan and heat, stirring periodically, for five minutes.

Mix in the salt, black pepper, turmeric, coriander, paprika, and ground cumin.

Include the vegetable broth, chopped tomatoes, and chickpeas. Once the sweet potatoes are cooked, simmer for 20 to 25 minutes on low heat after bringing to a boil.

Cook the kale or spinach for a further two to three minutes, or until it wilts.

Before serving, add lemon juice if preferred and adjust seasoning as necessary.

Barley Risotto with Mushrooms

(per serving, 1 cup):

Calories: 280

Protein: 10g

Fat: 8g

Carbs: 40g

Fiber: 6g

Calcium: 200 mg

Prep Time: 10 minutes Cooking Time: 35-40 minutes

1 cup pearl barley

1 tablespoon olive oil

1 small onion, finely chopped

2 cloves garlic, minced

1 cup mushrooms, sliced

4 cups low-sodium vegetable broth or chicken broth

1/2 cup dry white wine (optional)

1/2 cup grated Parmesan cheese

1/4 cup chopped fresh parsley

Salt and pepper

In a saucepan, warm the vegetable broth and maintain a low temperature.

Heat the olive oil in a big pan over medium heat. Add the onion and garlic, and sauté for 3 to 4 minutes, or until softened.

Add the mushrooms and simmer for about 5 minutes, or until they release their juices and become soft.

Add the pearl barley and simmer, stirring, for one to two minutes, until it starts to toast.

Add the white wine, if using, and heat it until the majority of it evaporates.

Start adding the heated broth with a ladle at a time, stirring regularly and letting it soak completely before Continue cooking for another 30 to 35 minutes, or until the barley is creamy and soft.

Add the Parmesan cheese and taste and adjust the seasoning. If desired, garnish with fresh parsley.

Whole Grain Couscous with Almonds

(per serving, 1 cup):

Calories: 250

Protein: 6g

Fat: 10g

Carbs: 34g

Fiber: 4g

Calcium: 80 mg

Prep Time: 10 minutes Cooking Time: 10 minutes

1 cup whole grain couscous

1 1/4 cups low-sodium vegetable broth or water

1/4 cup sliced almonds

1/4 cup chopped dried apricots

1 tablespoon olive oil

1/4 teaspoon ground cinnamon

1/4 cup fresh parsley, chopped

Salt and pepper

Bring the vegetable stock to a boil in a medium saucepan. Stir in the couscous, cover, and turn off the heat. After letting it settle for around five minutes, fluff with a fork.

In a small pan over medium heat, warm the olive oil while the couscous cooks. After adding the sliced almonds, roast them for 3 to 4 minutes, stirring often, until they become golden brown. Take caution not to scorch them.

Put the cooked couscous, chopped dried apricots, roasted almonds, and cinnamon (if using) in a big bowl. To taste, add salt and pepper for seasoning.

If wanted, garnish with fresh parsley. Heat or serve at room temperature.

Lentil and Quinoa Pilaf with Spinach

(per serving, 1 cup):

Calories: 250

Protein: 10g

Fat: 6g

Carbs: 36g

Fiber: 8g

Calcium: 80 mg

Prep Time: 10 minutes Cooking Time: 30 minutes

1/2 cup dried green or brown lentils

1/2 cup quinoa

1 small onion, finely chopped

2 cloves garlic, minced

1 tablespoon olive oil

1 cup vegetable or chicken broth

1 cup water

1 cup fresh spinach, chopped

1/2 teaspoon ground cumin

1/2 teaspoon paprika

Salt and pepper

1/4 cup chopped fresh parsley

Give the lentils a quick rinse in cold water. The lentils and one cup of water should be combined in a medium pot. After bringing to a boil, lower the heat, and simmer until soft, about 20 minutes. After removing any extra water, keep away.

Give the grain a quick rinse in cold water. Bring one cup of water and one cup of vegetable or chicken broth to a boil in a different pot. After adding the quinoa, lower the heat, cover, and simmer until the quinoa is cooked and the liquid has been absorbed—about 15 minutes. Using a fork, fluff and put aside.

Heat the olive oil in a big pan over medium heat. Add the chopped onion and simmer for approximately 5 minutes, or until softened. After adding the garlic, heat it for one more minute.

Transfer the quinoa and cooked lentils to the skillet. Add the paprika, ground cumin, salt, and pepper and stir. Cook for another five minutes, stirring now and again.

Cook the chopped spinach for two minutes, or until it wilts.

If wanted, top with freshly chopped parsley and serve warm.

Chickpea Salad with Cucumber, Tomato

(per serving, about 1 cup):

Calories: 250

Protein: 10g

Fat: 14g

Carbs: 25g

Fiber: 7g

Calcium: 80 mg

Prep Time: 10 minutes Cooking Time: None

1 can (15 oz) chickpeas, drained and rinsed

1 cup cucumber, diced

1 cup cherry tomatoes, halved

1/4 cup red onion, finely chopped

2 tablespoons extra virgin olive oil

1 tablespoon lemon juice or red wine vinegar

1/4 cup fresh parsley, chopped or basil

Salt and pepper

Put the chickpeas, cucumber, cherry tomatoes, and red onion (if using) in a big bowl.

Mix the lemon juice, olive oil, salt, and pepper in a small bowl.

Drizzle the dressing over the combination of chickpeas, tossing to cover well.

Add the chopped basil or parsley and stir.

To let the flavors mingle, enjoy right away or store in the refrigerator for 30 minutes.

Millet Porridge with Almonds

(per serving, 2 servings):

Calories: 270

Protein: 8g

Fat: 12g

Carbs: 34g

Fiber: 5g

Calcium: 150 mg

Prep Time: 10 minutes Cooking Time: 20 minutes

1 cup millet

2 1/2 cups water or low-fat milk

1/4 teaspoon salt

1 tablespoon honey or maple syrup

1/2 teaspoon vanilla extract

1/4 cup sliced almonds

1/2 cup fresh berries

Give the millet a good rinse in cold water.

Heat the milk or water to a boil in a medium saucepan. Stir in the salt and millet. After turning down the heat to low, cover, and simmer the millet for approximately 20 minutes, or until it is soft and the liquid has been absorbed.

Add vanilla essence, if used, and honey or maple syrup.

Ladle into bowls with the porridge. Spread some fresh berries and almond slices on top.

3: Exercise and Lifestyle Strategies for Bone Strength

The Role of Exercise in Bone Health

Exercises for Gaining Weight

Exercises involving weight bearing force you to move against gravity while maintaining your upright posture. Because they promote bone growth and slow down bone loss, these workouts are essential for preserving and increasing bone density. Important details about weight-bearing activities are as follows:

- High-Impact Weight-Bearing Exercises: These consist of aerobics, dancing, leaping, and running. They work very well to increase the density of bone in the legs, hips, and spine. They may not be appropriate for everyone, particularly for people who already have joint problems or bone disorders[1].
- Low-Impact Weight-Bearing Exercises: These include elliptical machine use, hiking, and brisk walking; they are kinder to the joints. They are a wonderful alternative for those who must refrain from high-impact activities and are advantageous for preserving bone density[1].

Workouts for Resistance

Strength training, or resistance exercise, is the practice of using your muscles to exert force against an outside force. The development and maintenance of muscle mass, which in turn supports and protects your bones, is made possible by these activities. The following are some crucial elements of resistance training:

- Free Weights and Machines: You may strengthen your bones and target certain muscle groups by using dumbbells, barbells, and weight machines. Squats, lunges, bench presses, and bicep curls are some of these exercises[1].

- Body Weight Exercises: Push-ups, pull-ups, and planks are among the exercises that utilize your own body weight as resistance. They work well without the use of equipment to increase bone and muscular strength1.
- Resistance Bands: These are tools with different resistance levels that are portable and adaptable. Resistance band exercises include shoulder presses, arm curls, and leg lifts1.

Combining Resistance and Weightlifting Exercises

It's crucial to include resistance and weight-bearing activities into your fitness regimen for the best possible bone health. Here are some pointers for mixing up these workouts:

- Balanced Routine: Try to include strength training two to three times per week and weight-bearing activities at least three to four times per week. This combination aids in maintaining muscle mass and promoting bone growth1.
- Variety: To target different muscle groups and avoid monotony, mix up your training routines. For instance, you can spend the week alternating between yoga, weightlifting, and running.
- Progressive Overload: To keep your bones and muscles challenged, progressively increase the time, intensity, and resistance of your workouts. This may include attempting more difficult exercises, raising the weight, or increasing the number of repetitions1.

Additional Advantages of Physical Activity for Bone Health

Frequent exercise helps reduce falls and fractures by strengthening the bones and improving balance, coordination, and flexibility. Additionally, it lowers the chance of developing chronic illnesses including osteoporosis, cardiovascular disease, and diabetes1. It also improves general health and wellbeing.

Bone Strengthening Exercise and Lifestyle Practices

Balance and Flexibility: Avoiding Falls

Preventing falls, which may result in fractures and other injuries, particularly in older persons, requires maintaining balance and flexibility. Stretching programs and other flexibility exercises assist maintain the limberness of muscles and joints, increasing range of motion and lowering the risk of injury. Exercises for balance enhance coordination and stability, both of which are necessary for keeping good posture and averting falls. Here are a few productive workouts:

- Heel-to-Toe Walk: Step forward with one foot exactly in front of the other's toes while maintaining a straight gait. This improves coordination and balance.
- Leg Raises: Raise one leg to the side while holding onto a chair for support. Lower it and switch to the other leg. The hips and outer thighs become stronger as a result.
- Calf Raises: Place your feet hip-width apart, raise your body to the tips of your toes, and then descend again. This builds muscle in the calves, which is important for balance.
- Tai Chi: With slow, deliberate motions, this soft, flowing workout enhances muscular strength, flexibility, and balance.

The Finest Activities to Increase Bone Density

Osteoporosis and fracture prevention depend on preserving and increasing bone density. Exercises involving weight bearing and resistance are very useful for this:

- Weight-Bearing Exercises: These consist of stair climbing, walking, running, dancing, and trekking. By making your body struggle against gravity, they promote the creation of new bones
- Resistance Training: Exercises like squats, lunges, push-ups, and weightlifting that use weights, resistance bands, or body weight may help strengthen bones and increase muscle mass
- High-Impact Activities: Because they place stronger stresses on the bones, exercises like running, leaping, and plyometrics have a bigger effect on bone strength.
- Yoga and Pilates: These workouts enhance bone health by enhancing muscular strength, flexibility, and balance.

Developing a Customized Workout Program

To optimize the advantages for bone health, an activity regimen customized to your individual requirements and objectives should be followed. The following actions may be taken to draft a winning plan:

- Assess Your Fitness Level: Recognize your present state of fitness, as well as your advantages, disadvantages, and potential restrictions. Your strategy will be guided by this self-awareness
- Set Clear Goals: Identify your objectives, such as boosting general fitness, improving balance, or improving bone density

- Incorporate Variety: To address multiple areas of bone health[3], use a variety of weight-bearing, resistance, flexibility, and balance activities.
- Schedule Regular Workouts: At least twice a week should be dedicated to muscle-strengthening activities. Aim for 150 minutes of moderate-intensity exercise or 75 minutes of high-intensity exercise per week
- Progress Gradually: Begin with exercises that correspond to your fitness level and progressively increase the intensity, duration, and resistance to continue challenging your bones and muscles.
- Remain Consistent: Maintaining consistency is essential to reaping long-term rewards. To keep your routine interesting and productive, follow it and tweak it as necessary

Bone Health and Sleep

The Significance of Healing Sleep

Healthy sleep is essential for maintaining overall health, which includes strong bones. The body goes through vital functions including tissue development, protein synthesis, and muscle repair during deep sleep and REM (rapid eye movement) sleep6. The body produces bone and muscle, heals and regrows tissues, and fortifies the immune system throughout these sleep stages1. Insufficient sleep may raise cortisol levels, which can eventually damage bones by causing the body to remove calcium from them1. Getting 7-8 hours of good sleep per night is essential for keeping your bones healthy.

Tips for Better Sleep Hygiene for Stronger Bones

Maintaining good sleep hygiene may greatly enhance the quality of your sleep, which will promote the health of your bones. Here are some pointers:

- Maintain a Consistent Sleep Schedule: Even on weekends, go to bed and get up at the same time each day. This aids in regulating the internal clock of your body
- Optimize Your Sleep Environment: Make sure your bedroom is cold, dark, and quiet before bed.
- Create a Relaxing Bedtime Routine: Read before bed, take a warm bath, or practice meditation.
- Exercise Regularly: Regular exercise can help you fall asleep faster and enjoy deeper sleep.
- Avoid Heavy Meals and Alcohol: Eating large meals or drinking alcohol before bed can disrupt sleep patterns.

- Limit Stimulants: Avoid caffeine and nicotine close to bedtime as they can interfere with your ability to fall asleep. But stay away from strenuous exertion just before bed.

Tackling Osteoporosis and Sleep Disorders

Because they interfere with sleep patterns and decrease the quantity of restorative sleep that occurs, sleep disorders including insomnia, sleep apnea, and restless leg syndrome may have a detrimental effect on bone health. The following are some methods for treating these conditions:

- Insomnia: Cognitive-behavioral therapy for insomnia (CBT-I) is an effective treatment that helps transform attitudes and behaviors that create or aggravate sleep problems
- Sleep Apnea: By keeping the airways open while you sleep, continuous positive airway pressure (CPAP) treatment is a standard technique to treat sleep apnea.
- Medication and lifestyle modifications, such cutting down on alcohol and caffeine, may help control symptoms of Restless Leg Syndrome.

Taking care of sleep disturbances is crucial for people with osteoporosis since insufficient sleep may worsen bone loss. Sleeping on your side with a cushion between your knees or on your back with a pillow beneath your knees are two examples of proper sleeping postures that may help reduce pain and enhance the quality of your sleep.

Melatonin's Function in Bone Density

A hormone best recognized for controlling sleep, melatonin is also important for bone health. Osteoblast activity, which is responsible for forming new bone, is stimulated, while osteoclast activity, which is responsible for reabsorbing existing bone, is inhibited. This process helps to create new bones. Research has shown that supplementing with melatonin might enhance bone mineral density, especially in women who have gone through menopause. Further promoting bone health are the antioxidant qualities of melatonin, which lessen oxidative stress on bone cells.

For optimal bone health, include foods high in melatonin, such tomatoes, grapes, and cherries, or think about taking melatonin supplements (under a doctor's supervision).

Sunlight and Bone Health

Sun Exposure and the Synthesis of Vitamin D

Because it facilitates the body's absorption of calcium, which is necessary for healthy bones, vitamin D is vital for bone health. Sunlight is the main source of vitamin D. The sun's ultraviolet B (UVB) rays cause your skin to change from a cholesterol derivative into vitamin D3 (cholecalciferol). The liver and kidneys subsequently convert this vitamin D3 into its active form, which the body may utilize. The amount of vitamin D your body makes from sun exposure depends on a number of factors, including skin pigmentation, age, location, and season.

Responsible Suncare Techniques for Ideal Bone Health

Even while exposure to sunshine is good for the production of vitamin D, it's crucial to practice safe sun exposure to prevent skin damage and lower the chance of skin cancer. Here are some pointers for sensible sun safety:

1. Timing: Try to get 10-15 minutes of sun exposure many times a week, ideally in the middle of the day when UVB rays are most beneficial for the synthesis of vitamin D.
2. Skin Protection: When spending prolonged amounts of time outside, use protective clothing, such as caps and long sleeves, and apply sunscreen to areas that are prone to sunburn.
3. Avoid Overexposure: Take care not to burn, particularly during the hours of greatest sunshine. Gradual exposure works better and is safer.
4. Individual Factors: When calculating the required quantity of sun exposure, take into account your skin type, age, and geographic region. Individuals with lighter skin tones manufacture vitamin D at a faster rate than those with darker skin tones[1].

Substitutes for Sunlight: Diet and Supplements

Supplements and food sources may support healthy vitamin D levels in those who get little sun exposure or who are susceptible to vitamin D deficiency:

- Supplements: Ergocalciferol (D2) and cholecalciferol (D3) are the two forms of vitamin D that are available as supplements. Vitamin D3 is superior at increasing and maintaining blood levels of vitamin D2. It's crucial to speak with a healthcare professional to figure out the right dose

- Nutritional Resources: Eat more foods high in vitamin D, such as egg yolks, fortified dairy products, fatty fish (salmon, mackerel, sardines), and fortified plant-based milks [3]. Most of the vitamin D in the diet comes from fortified foods, particularly in areas with little sunlight.

Light Therapy's Role

Artificial light is used in light treatment, commonly referred to as phototherapy, to simulate natural sunshine. Seasonally Affective Disorder (SAD) sufferers and those with little sun exposure will benefit most from this treatment. Sitting next to a bright light box that produces light, generally in the blue or white spectrum, for 20 to 30 minutes every morning is the standard protocol for light treatment. This exposure improves mood and sleep patterns by regulating serotonin and melatonin levels. Additionally, for those who are unable to obtain enough sunshine, light treatment may enhance bone health by encouraging the synthesis of vitamin D.

Keeping an Eye on Your Bone Health

Expectation of Bone Density Testing

An essential technique for identifying osteoporosis and determining fracture risk is bone density testing, which is often carried out using a dual-energy X-ray absorptiometry (DXA) scan. The test quantifies the calcium and other mineral content of a bone section, usually the forearm, hip, or spine. It's a short, painless, non-invasive process. A comfortable table will be used for you to lay on while a scanner scans your body. Radiation exposure is negligible—less than that of a typical chest X-ray5. The test results provide a T-score that shows whether you have normal bone density, osteopenia, or osteoporosis. The results also assist in identifying your bone density and compare it to the average bone density of a healthy young adult.

Monitoring Development: From Nutrition to Exercise

There's more to keeping an eye on your bone health than simply getting regular bone density testing. It's important to monitor your food and activity habits if you want to preserve and enhance your bone health. Here are a few ways to monitor your advancement:

- Diet: Keep a food journal to make sure you are receiving enough calcium, vitamin D, and other minerals that are good for your bones. You can track your daily consumption and keep an eye on your nutritional goals with the aid of apps like MyFitnessPal.

- Exercise: Record your physical activity using fitness trackers or apps. Keep track of the kinds of activities you do, including resistance and weight-bearing exercises, as well as their length and intensity1. Reviewing this data on a regular basis can help you modify your routines to optimize the advantages to bone health
- Body Measurements: Take regular measurements of your height, weight, and body composition. Record the results. Improvements in bone density and muscle mass may be indicated by changes in these metrics1.

Knowing Your Bone Health Ratings

T-scores and Z-scores are often used to report the results of bone density tests:

- T-score: This indicates how your bone density stacks up against that of a 30-year-old, healthy adult. A T-score between +1 and -1 is regarded as normal, between -1 and -2.5 as osteopenia (poor bone density), and between -2.5 and below as osteoporosis.
- Z-score: This indicates how much bone density is normal for your age, sex, and size. If the Z-score is less than -2.0, it might indicate that the cause of aberrant bone loss is not ageing.

Knowing these scores enables you and your healthcare practitioner to make well-informed choices about the management and potential treatments for your bone health.

When to Speak with an Expert

It is recommended that you see a specialist, such as an endocrinologist or rheumatologist, if you have osteoporosis risk factors or if the results of your bone density test show severe bone loss. In the following situations, you need to think about seeing a specialist:

- Unexplained Bone Loss: If you have a considerable drop in bone density without a clear explanation, a professional may assist in determining any underlying conditions.
- Fractures: If you sustain fractures from small trauma, your bones may be weakened and need more testing and care.
- Medication Management: A specialist can assist in managing the effects of drugs, such as steroids, on your bones
- Complex Cases: A specialist can offer comprehensive care and coordinate treatment plans if you have various health conditions that are impacting your bones.

Medication and Supplements

The Supplemental Function in Bone Health

Taking supplements may be very important for preserving and enhancing bone health, particularly in cases when food consumption is inadequate. The following are important nutrients for bone health: zinc, calcium, magnesium, vitamin K, and vitamin D. Together, these nutrients assist the synthesis, upkeep, and repair of bones

- Calcium: A necessary mineral for strong, well-formed bones. It is essential for preserving bone density and is the principal mineral present in bones
- Vitamin D: Promotes optimal intestinal absorption of calcium and sustains sufficient levels of phosphate and calcium in the blood for proper bone mineralization
- Magnesium: Contributes to bone production and regulates osteoblast and osteoclast activity (the cells that build and resorb bone).
- Vitamin K: Assists in the binding of calcium to the bone matrix and is involved in bone metabolism.
- Zinc: Vital for mineralization and the regeneration of bone tissue.

Use of Vitamin D and Calcium Supplements Safely

Even while supplements have several advantages, it's crucial to utilize them responsibly to prevent any negative effects and interactions:

- Calcium Supplements: Adults typically need 1,000–1,200 mg of calcium daily, while recommendations vary by age and gender1. Although dietary sources of calcium are preferable, supplements may help make up for any shortfall. Common types include calcium citrate and carbonate. While calcium citrate may be taken either way2, it is best to take calcium carbonate with meals for optimal absorption.
- Vitamin D Supplements: For most individuals, a daily dose of 600–800 IU of vitamin D is advised2. When it comes to increasing blood levels of vitamin D, vitamin D3 (cholecalciferol) is more efficient than vitamin D2 (ergocalciferol). It's crucial to follow a doctor's advice and not go above the daily maximum of 4,000 IU of vitamin D since this may result in toxicity.

Comprehending Drugs for Osteoporosis

To strengthen bones and lower the risk of fracture, a number of drugs are available to treat and prevent osteoporosis. These drugs function in various ways.

- Bisphosphonates: These medications, which include risedronate (Actonel) and alendronate (Fosamax), slow down bone loss and promote bone density.
- Selective Estrogen Receptor Modulators (SERMs): Raloxifene (Evista) mimics the positive effects of estrogen on bone density while avoiding some of the risks connected with estrogen therapy
- Hormone Replacement Therapy (HRT): Since estrogen therapy carries some risks, it is typically only advised for women who have noticeable menopausal symptoms
- Parathyroid Hormone Analogues: Teriparatide (Forteo) increases the formation of new bone and is used to treat severe osteoporosis
- RANK Ligand (RANKL) Inhibitors: Denosumab (Prolia) inhibits osteoclast activity to assist prevent bone resorption.

Natural Curatives and Complementary Therapies

Apart from traditional therapies, there are natural medicines and complementary therapies that may promote bone health:

- Herbal Supplements: Although there is little scientific proof, herbs including horsetail, black cohosh, and red clover are said to promote bone health.
- Isoflavones: Occurring in soy-based goods, isoflavones resemble estrogen and may aid in maintaining bone density
- Living Adjustments: A balanced diet high in nutrients that support strong bones, frequent weight-bearing exercise, and abstaining from tobacco and excessive alcohol use may all have a major positive influence on bone health.
- Tai Chi and acupuncture: By enhancing balance and lowering the risk of falls, these techniques may indirectly promote bone health

Bone Health at Various Stages of Life

Although preserving healthy bones is a lifetime responsibility, a person's age and stage of life have a considerable impact on the problems they face. Menopause and older adulthood are two crucial life stages that need extra care to preserve bone density and reduce the risk of osteoporosis.

Value of Strong Bones in Adolescence and Early Adulthood

The adolescent and early adult years are crucial for the development of bones. People attain their peak bone mass during these years, which is the highest point at which the strength and density of their bones may be achieved. By the age of 20 to 30´, this maximal bone mass is usually reached.

The incidence of osteoporosis and fractures later in life is inversely correlated with peak bone mass. To maintain healthy bones for the rest of one's life, it is crucial to pay attention to bone health throughout these formative years.

Maintaining Bone Density during Menopause

Every woman will naturally go through the menopause, which usually happens around the age of 50. Nonetheless, it has a significant effect on bone health. The menopause results in a significant reduction in estrogen levels, which is a hormone that is necessary for preserving bone density. This decrease in estrogen speeds up the deterioration of bone, which often results in a sharp decline in bone mass in the years just after menopause. This may be the start of a higher risk of osteoporosis for many women.

Recognizing Estrogen's Function in Bone Health

The balance between the production of new bone and the breakdown of existing bone is largely dependent on estrogen. Estrogen aids in controlling the activity of osteoclasts, the cells that tear down bone tissue, throughout the reproductive years. By controlling the pace of bone deterioration, it promotes the formation of new bone tissue and preserves bone density.

This equilibrium is upset after menopause when estrogen levels decline. Increased osteoclast activity causes more bone to be broken down than to be rebuilt. Because of this, women may lose as much as 20% of their bone density in the first five to seven years after menopause, increasing their risk of fractures, particularly those involving the wrists, hips, and spine.

Important Techniques for Preserving Bone Density during Menopause

1. Make calcium and vitamin D intake a priority:

The two most important nutrients for healthy bones are calcium and vitamin D, especially after menopause. The main component of bone tissue is calcium, and vitamin D facilitates the body's more effective absorption of calcium.

The daily recommended calcium intake rises to around 1,200 mg throughout menopause. Foods high in calcium, such as dairy products, leafy greens, fortified plant milks, and fish with bones, such salmon and sardines, should be consumed by women.

Vitamin D has similar significance. Insufficient amounts of this vitamin may make it difficult to maintain bone density, even with a diet high in calcium. The greatest natural source of vitamin D is sunshine exposure, however many women may need to take supplements to get the 600–800 IU of vitamin D they need daily, depending on their lifestyle and place of residence.

2. Include Resistance and Weight Training Exercises:

Frequent exercise is essential for preserving bone mass both during and after menopause. Weight-bearing activities push on the bones, promoting the development of new bones, such as walking, running, and dancing. By strengthening the muscles that surround bones, resistance activities like weightlifting and resistance band use may lower the risk of fractures and falls.

Maintaining bone health requires doing strength-training and weight-bearing workouts at least three times each week. Exercises that enhance balance and coordination, such as tai chi or yoga, may also help lower the risk of falls, which are a major factor in fractures in women going through menopause.

3. Take into Account Hormone Replacement Treatment (HRT):

One kind of medication that helps lessen the bone loss brought on by menopause is hormone replacement therapy (HRT). HRT may help decrease the pace of bone loss and, in some situations, even restore bone density by restoring estrogen levels. HRT is not risk-free, however, so it's crucial for every woman to speak with her doctor and consider the advantages and possible drawbacks—which might include a higher chance of developing certain cancers and heart problems.

Other drugs like bisphosphonates or selective estrogen receptor modulators (SERMs) may be provided to women who are unable to use HRT or who want not to in order to assist maintain bone density.

4. Give Your Diet a Balance:

Apart from calcium and vitamin D, a balanced diet is crucial for maintaining bone health during menopause. Vitamin K2, potassium, and magnesium-rich foods all help to maintain bone density. Nuts, seeds, whole grains, and leafy greens are good sources of magnesium. Whole foods high in potassium, such as sweet potatoes and bananas, may help balance the body's acidic pH, which weakens bones.

One important function of vitamin K2, which is included in fermented foods and certain animal products, is to prevent calcium from building up in the arteries and instead going straight to the bones and teeth.

5. Steer clear of excessive alcohol and smoking:

Bone loss may be caused by smoking and binge drinking too much alcohol. Drinking alcohol may lower bone growth and raise the risk of falls, while smoking affects estrogen levels and the body's capacity to absorb calcium. Menopausal women should abstain from all tobacco products and restrict their alcohol consumption to one drink per day.

Senior Bone Health: Particular Considerations

Due to the natural lowering of bone density with age, elderly are more susceptible to osteoporosis and fractures. In actuality, one in five men and one in three women over 50 will have an osteoporosis-related fracture. Even while some bone density loss is normal with age, seniors may still use effective measures to preserve bone strength and lower their risk of crippling fractures.

Comprehending Bone Loss Associated with Age

Around age 30, bone mass peaks and then progressively decreases. Usually, by the time a person reaches their senior years, their bone density has greatly decreased, particularly if they did not take aggressive measures to maintain bone health earlier in life.

Other age-related variables, such as decreased physical activity, lower levels of vitamin D from less sun exposure, and poor calcium absorption, often exacerbate the loss of bone density in seniors. Seniors are also more prone to fall because of diminished muscle mass, eyesight problems, and poor balance, which raises their risk of fracture.

Techniques for Preserving Elderly Bone Health

Make Sure you're Eating Enough Nutrients:

The demand for calcium and vitamin D increases much higher for elderly people. For a variety of reasons, such as reduced appetite, restricted availability to fresh foods, or lactose intolerance, many older persons may find it difficult to get adequate calcium from their diet alone. To get the daily recommended consumption of 1,200 milligrams of calcium, it may be essential to take supplements, under the supervision of a healthcare expert.

Seniors need vitamin D just as much since their skin is less capable of absorbing it from sunshine. Aim for 800–1,000 IU of vitamin D per day for seniors, either from fortified foods or supplements.

Use Exercise to Prevent Falls:

Retaining balance and mobility is essential for elder fall prevention. Walking and other weight-bearing exercises are still vital, but those with joint discomfort or mobility limitations may benefit more from low-impact sports like cycling and swimming. Strength training is especially crucial for preserving muscle mass and stabilizing the bones, which lowers the chance of fractures.

Exercises for balance, like yoga or standing on one leg, are crucial for lowering the risk of falls. To keep their joints in their full range of motion, seniors can also focus on improving their flexibility.

Increasing Home Safety:

Fall prevention is important for seniors, and there are many things that can be done to lower the chance of falls at home. A safer atmosphere may be produced by adding grab bars to toilets, minimizing trip hazards like loose carpets, making sure there is enough lighting, and using non-slip matting. Seniors should also have frequent checks on their hearing and vision since these senses may be compromised and lead to falls.

Bone Health Medication:

Medications such as bisphosphonates, denosumab, or teriparatide may be provided to seniors who have osteoporosis and are at high risk of fractures in order to decrease bone loss and, in some situations, restore bone density. Seniors and their healthcare professionals should collaborate carefully to assess the efficacy and adverse effects of these drugs.

Bone health and social support:

Keeping up social ties becomes crucial for general health, especially bone health, as elders become older. Loneliness and isolation may result in depression, which can lower desire to practice good habits like working out or eating well. Seniors may maintain their bone health habits by participating in group fitness courses, attending community activities, and receiving encouragement from their families.

APPENDICES

7 DAY MEAL PLAN

Day 1:

Breakfast: Oatmeal with Ground Flax Seeds (27)
Lunch: Spinach and Feta Omelette (16)
Dinner: Baked Trout with Lemon and Garlic (59)
Snack: Almonds and Dried Figs (36)

Day 2:

Breakfast: Fortified Cereal with Milk and Banana (28)
Lunch: Quinoa Salad with Spinach, Chickpeas, and Feta (85)
Dinner: Baked Chicken Thighs with Garlic (53)
Snack: Cottage Cheese with Pineapple (12)

Day 3:

Breakfast: Smoothie Bowl with Fortified Soy Milk (30)
Lunch: Sardines on Whole-Grain Toast (54)
Dinner: Black Bean and Sweet Potato Enchiladas (66)
Snack: Kale Chips (39)

Day 4:

Breakfast: Egg Muffins with Spinach and Cheese (21)
Lunch: Lentil Soup with Kale and Carrots (86)
Dinner: Salmon and Avocado on Whole-Grain Toast (20)
Snack: Fortified Almond Milk Latte (38)

Day 5:

Breakfast: Buckwheat Pancakes with Walnuts (34)
Lunch: Chickpea Salad with Cucumber, Tomato (99)
Dinner: Mackerel with Olive Oil and Roasted Vegetables (55)
Snack: String Cheese with Grapes (40)

Day 6:

Breakfast: Tofu Scramble with Spinach (18)
Lunch: Whole Wheat Pita with Hummus and Cucumber (71)
Dinner: Lamb Chops with Kale and Sweet Potatoes (51)
Snack: Mixed Berry and Spinach Smoothie (44)

Day 7:

Breakfast: Ricotta and Berry Toast on Whole Grain Bread (15)
Lunch: Tuna Salad with Spinach and Avocado (60)
Dinner: Chickpea and Sweet Potato Stew (92)
Snack: Fortified Soy Yogurt with Fresh Berries (80)

Frequently Asked Questions (FAQs)

1. Define osteoporosis

Osteoporosis is characterized by weak and brittle bones that are more likely to fracture. It happens when the body loses too much bone mass, produces too little bone, or both, resulting in decreased bone density.

2. What are some early indicators of osteoporosis?

Osteoporosis is commonly referred to as a "silent disease" since it does not produce evident symptoms until a bone fractures. Early warning signals might include:
   Symptoms may include loss of height, a stooped posture, back discomfort from a collapsed or broken vertebra, and fragile bones that readily shatter with simple falls or traumas.

3. What are the risk factors for getting osteoporosis?

Several factors may raise the risk of osteoporosis, including:
  - Age: Bone density normally diminishes with age.
  - Gender: Women have a higher risk of developing osteoporosis, especially after menopause.
  - Family history: A family history of osteoporosis raises your risk.
  - Inadequate calcium and vitamin D intake: Poor bone nutrition deteriorates bones over time.
  - Sedentary lifestyle: A lack of physical exercise might lower bone strength.
  - Smoking and heavy alcohol consumption: Both may lead to bone loss.

4. Why is bone health essential for all ages?

Maintaining bone health is essential at all stages of life. Your body accumulates bone mass between infancy and adolescence, reaching a peak around the age of 30. After that, you begin to lose bone mass, so maintaining a healthy lifestyle, including a calcium-rich diet and weight-bearing activity, is critical for slowing bone loss and preventing osteoporosis.

5. How can nutrition influence bone health?
Diet has an important influence in bone health. Consuming enough calcium, vitamin D, magnesium, and potassium promotes bone density. A shortage of essential nutrients weakens bones, making them more prone to fractures.

6. Which foods help to keep healthy bones?

Foods high in calcium, vitamin D, and other bone-building minerals include:
  - Dairy products, including milk, yogurt, and cheese.
  - Leafy greens, including kale, spinach, and bok choy
  - Fish such as salmon and sardines (particularly with bones)
  - fortified foods, such as plant-based milk and orange juice.
  - Nuts, seeds, and legumes, including almonds, chia seeds, and chickpeas

7. What are some calcium-rich non-dairy foods?

Non Dairy calcium sources include:
  - Leafy greens (such as kale and collard greens).
  - Fortified plant-based milk (such as almond, soy, or oat milk)
  Tofu and tempeh.
  - Almonds and sesame seeds.
  - Broccoli with Bok Choy
  - Sardines and salmon with bones.

8. How does menopause influence bone health?

During menopause, estrogen levels decline considerably, hastening bone loss. Women may lose up to 20% of their bone density in the first 5-7 years after menopause. During and after menopause, it is critical to prioritize bone health via nutrition, exercise, and, in certain cases, medications.

9. How can lifestyle modifications help prevent or treat osteoporosis?

Key lifestyle adjustments to prevent or treat osteoporosis are:
  - Consuming a balanced diet rich in calcium and vitamin D.
  - Engaging in regular weight. Weight-bearing and muscle-strengthening workouts, such as walking, running, or lifting weights
  - Avoid smoking and heavy alcohol intake.
  - Getting frequent bone density examinations (particularly for women after menopause).
  - Taking calcium and vitamin D supplements as needed, according to your doctor's instructions

10. How much calcium and vitamin D should I consume daily?

The recommended daily consumption varies by age and gender.
  - Adults under 50: 1,000 mg calcium and 400-800 IU vitamin D.
  - Adults 50 and older: 1,200 mg calcium and 800-1,000 IU vitamin D.
  These levels may be altered depending on personal health requirements or medical advice.

11. What are the greatest workouts for increasing bone strength?

Weight-bearing and resistance activities are the most effective in maintaining and increasing bone density. This includes:
  - Physical activities such as walking, running, and hiking - Strength training using weights and resistance bands
  - Yoga or Pilates (flexibility and balance)
  - Dancing or Aerobics
  These activities encourage bone regeneration and strengthen the muscles around the bones, lowering the risk of falls and fractures.

12. Is osteoporosis preventable?

While certain risk factors, including heredity and age, cannot be avoided, osteoporosis may often be prevented or postponed with a healthy lifestyle. Regular exercise, a calcium and vitamin D-rich diet, quitting smoking, and limiting alcohol use may all help to minimize your chance of developing osteoporosis.

13. Can males have osteoporosis?

Yes, males may get osteoporosis, although it is more frequent in women. Men normally lose bone mass later in life than women, but by the age of 65 or 70, they lose bone density at the same pace. Men with low testosterone levels, heavy drinkers, and those on particular drugs may be at an increased risk.

14. Should I use calcium or vitamin D supplements?

If you don't receive enough calcium or vitamin D from your diet, your doctor may suggest supplements. It is critical not to exceed the recommended daily calcium intake, since too much calcium might result in kidney stones and other health problems. Before beginning any supplement regimen, always speak with your doctor.

15. How does vitamin K influence bone health?

Vitamin K regulates calcium and improves bone health by activating the proteins required for bone mineralization. Leafy greens such as kale, spinach, and broccoli are rich in vitamin K.

16. Is osteoporosis reversible?

Osteoporosis cannot be completely reversed, but it may be treated to prevent additional bone loss. You may enhance bone strength and minimize your risk of fractures by following a healthy diet, exercising regularly, using medications, and other lifestyle changes.

17. What is a bone density test, and when should I get it?

A bone density examination, or DEXA scan, determines the strength and density of your bones. It's a rapid and non-invasive exam. Bone density testing is normally suggested for women over 65 and males over 70. People with risk factors (such as a family history or early menopause) should see their doctor about being tested sooner.

18. What drugs are used to treat osteoporosis?

There are many drugs available for treating osteoporosis, including:
- Bisphosphonates: slows bone loss and fracture risk.
- Denosumab: Injectable medicine that slows bone resorption.
- Hormone therapy: Replaces estrogen in postmenopausal women.
- Parathyroid hormone (PTH) analogs: Promotes new bone development.

Always talk with your healthcare practitioner to decide the best treatment plan for you.

19. Are osteoporosis-related fractures serious?

Yes, fractures caused by osteoporosis may be quite dangerous, especially hip fractures, which often need surgery and lengthy recovery times. Spinal fractures may cause persistent discomfort, height loss, and a stooped posture, all of which have a substantial influence on quality of life.

20. How can I determine whether I'm at risk for osteoporosis?

If you are over 50 and have had a bone fracture, have a family history of osteoporosis, are postmenopausal or have undergone early menopause, or have a low body weight or a tiny body frame, you may be at risk of developing osteoporosis.
   - Use drugs like corticosteroids long-term.
   If you believe you are at risk, speak with your doctor about obtaining a bone density test and techniques for maintaining bone health.

RECIPE INDEX

Q

Quinoa Porridge with Almond Butter33
Quinoa Salad with Spinach, Chickpeas, and Feta85

R

Ricotta and Berry Toast on Whole Grain Bread15

S

Sardines on Whole-Grain Toast54
Shrimp Stir-Fry with Bok Choy57
Spinach and Feta Omelette16
Salmon and Avocado on Whole-Grain Toast20
Sweet Potato Hash with Poached Eggs23
Smoothie Bowl with Fortified Soy Milk30
Sardines on Whole Grain Crackers31
String Cheese with Grapes40
Sardines on Whole Wheat Crackers41

T

Tofu Scramble with Spinach18
Turkey Chili with Beans49
Tuna Salad with Spinach and Avocado60
Tofu Scramble with Spinach75

V

Vegan Sweet Potato and Black Bean Tacos76
Vegan Lentil Soup with Spinach and Carrots78
Vegan Whole Grain Toast with Avocado81

W

Whole Wheat Waffles with Greek Yogurt13
Whole Wheat Pita with Hummus and Cucumber71

Made in United States
Orlando, FL
11 November 2024

53724107R00070